Cytokines in Transfusion Medicine: A Primer

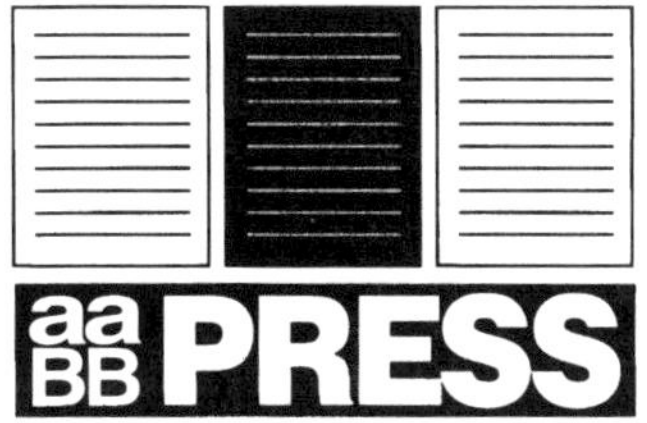

Cytokines in Transfusion Medicine: A Primer

Editors

Robertson D. Davenport, MD
University of Michigan Medical School
Ann Arbor, Michigan

Edward L. Snyder, MD
Yale University School of Medicine
Yale-New Haven Hospital
New Haven, Connecticut

AABB Press
Bethesda, Maryland
1997

American Association of Blood Banks
8101 Glenbrook Road
Bethesda, Maryland 20814-2749

ISBN NO. 1-56395-080-4
Printed in the United States

Library of Congress Cataloging-in-Publication Data

Cytokines in transfusion medicine: a primer/editors, Robertson D. Davenport, Edward L. Snyder.
p. cm.
Includes bibliographical references and index.
ISBN 1-56395-080-4 (hardbound)
1.Blood—Transfusion—Complications. 2. Cytokines—Pathophysiology.
3. Biological response modifiers—Pathophysiology.
I. Davenport, Robertson D. II. Snyder, Edward L. (Edward Leonard), 1946-.
[DNLM: 1. Cytokines—physiology. 2. Biological Response Modifiers—physiology.
3. Blood Transfusion. QW 568 C9964345 1997]
RM171.C98 1997
615' .39—dc21
DNLM/DLC
for Library of Congress

97-35729
CIP

AABB Press Editorial Board

Contributors

David Berkowicz, MD, MSC
Laboratory of Computer Science
Massachusetts General Hospital
Boston, Massachusetts

Robertson D. Davenport, MD
University of Michigan Blood Bank
Ann Arbor, Michigan

Stephen G. Emerson, MD, PhD
University of Pennsylvania School of Medicine
Philadelphia, Pennsylvania

Terrence L. Geiger, MD, PhD
Yale University School of Medicine
New Haven, Connecticut

Raza A. Khan, MD
University of Michigan
Ann Arbor, Michigan

Steven L. Kunkel, PhD
The University of Michigan Medical School
Ann Arbor, Michigan

Susan F. Leitman, MD
Warren G. Magnuson Clinical Center
Bethesda, Maryland

Marian Petrides, MD
University of Mississippi Medical Center
Jackson, Mississippi

John W. Smith II, MD
Earle A. Chiles Research Institute
Portland, Oregon

Edward L. Snyder, MD
Yale University School of Medicine
New Haven, Connecticut

Gary Stack, MD, PhD
VA Medical Center
West Haven, Connecticut

David F. Stroncek, MD
Warren G. Magnuson Clinical Center
Bethesda, Maryland

Table of Contents

Preface

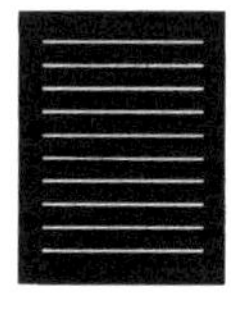

WHEN WE TRANSFUSE BLOOD WE ARE TRYING TO DO more than elevate cell counts or factor levels; we are trying to achieve a biologic response. The desired biologic response may be an increase in tissue oxygenation, the prevention of hemorrhage, or the cessation of bleeding. Of course, unfavorable biologic responses may also occur, such as fever, hypotension, immune suppression, or acute lung injury. As the field of blood banking has evolved into transfusion medicine, we have come increasingly to recognize the need to focus on biologic responses to blood transfusion and the factors that influence such responses.

Blood transfusion is the prototypical and most frequently performed transplantation procedure. Transfusion not only introduces alloantigens to a recipient, but also metabolically active cells. These cells may be capable of persisting in the recipient by proliferating and responding to stimuli from the host and producing response modifiers that affect the recipient. In addition, as blood components are collected, processed, and stored, donor cells may be stimulated to produce response modifiers. Finally, the recipient will frequently respond to the challenge of transfusion by producing mediators of the immune and inflammatory responses that further influence the patient's clinical response. Biological response modifiers encompass a broad range of molecules produced by donor or recipient cells that influence the clinical response to blood transfusion. These response modifiers can be grouped into three general categories. The first category includes molecules that are in an inactive precursor form in plasma, such as components of the complement and kinin systems. These modifiers do not require cellular events to be converted into an active form. The anaphylotoxins C3a, C4a, and C5a, for instance, are released from complement components by specific convertase enzyme complexes. Similarly, bradykinin is a product of the enzymatic cleavage of high molecular weight kininogen.

The second category of response modifiers encompasses products of cellular activation, which include the cytokines, growth factors, nitric oxide, and the prostaglandins. The production of these factors requires metabolic activity, and in the case of most cytokines, gene transcription and mRNA translation. Transfused donor leukocytes and recipient cells may be sources of such factors. Since active cellular processes are required for the production of these factors, a great range of biologic responses is possible.

The last general category of biological response modifiers are preformed, packaged factors that are released upon cellular activation. Examples of this class include the cytokine RANTES and platelet factor 4, which are present in platelet alpha granules. These response modifiers share some of the characteristics of the first two categories, but are previously synthesized and sequestered within cells. Cellular processes are required for their release; however, gene expression is not. Transfusion reactions are prime examples of how biological response modifiers may alter the outcome of blood transfusion. The clinical manifestations of hemolytic transfusion reactions are the direct result of the release of soluble complement components and the production of cytokines by stimulated phagocytes. Febrile nonhemolytic transfusion reactions are a consequence of the recipient production of pyrogenic cytokines and the in vitro production of the same substances by donor leukocytes during blood component storage. The occurrence and course of such reactions are dependent on the precise amount and type of cytokines involved.

Biological response modifiers may also have salutary effects on blood transfusion recipients. Principally, the hematopoietic growth factors are having a considerable impact on the practice of blood transfusion. Erythropoietin historically was the first, which has dramatically altered red cell transfusion requirements in patients with renal failure. Increasingly, other growth factors such as IL-11 and GM-CSF are changing the transfusion requirements and outcomes of patients with chemotherapy-induced myelosuppression and in bone marrow transplantation. Hematopoietic growth factors are also having a more limited but increasing impact on blood and progenitor cell donation.

This book provides an introduction to the roles of cytokines and biological response modifiers in transfusion medicine. The first chapter provides an overview of the cellular production and effects of cytokines as well as classification and terminology. The second chapter reviews the increasingly important problems of cytokine production by cellular blood components during storage and their clinical effects on transfusion recipients. Continuing on the theme of the previous chapter, Chapter 3 addresses the production of biologic response modifiers, including cytokines and complement components, that occur during the processing of blood components. The complex interactions of these biological mediators and leukocyte-reduction filters are also discussed. In the fourth chapter, the pivotal role of inflammatory cytokines, chemokines, and anti-inflammatory cytokines in the pathophysiology of hemolytic transfusion reaction is discussed.

In three related chapters, Chapters 5, 6, and 7, the biology and clinical application of hematopoietic growth factors in transfusion medicine are discussed. The first of these chapters focuses on erythropoietin and the production of red blood cells. The second chapter covers biology and clinical effects of leukocyte growth factors, with particular reference to the use of these agents in peripheral blood hematopoietic stem cell harvesting. Emerging results from basic science and clinical trials relating to the stimulation of platelet production by cytokines and hematopoietic growth factors are discussed in third chapter of this group. The final chapter, which is closely related to the previous three, discusses the role of hematopoietic growth factors and other cytokines in the rapidly developing field of ex-vivo expansion of blood progenitor cells.

The fields of inflammatory mediators, cytokines, and hematopoietic growth factors are vast and rapidly expanding. We make no pretense of completeness. Rather, in this book we are attempting to bring together different aspects of biological response modifiers as they pertain to transfusion medicine in order to develop common themes. We hope that through this book, the reader will develop a general understanding of how these diverse and potent molecules are shaping clinical responses to blood transfusion and the field of transfusion medicine itself.

Robertson D. Davenport, MD
Edward L. Snyder, MD
Editors

About the Editors

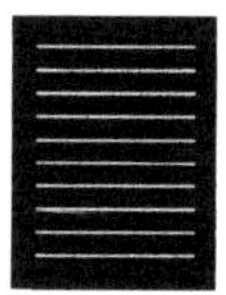

Robertson D. Davenport, MD, is Associate Professor of Pathology at the University of Michigan Medical School, and Associate Medical Director of the Blood Bank and Transfusion Service of the University of Michigan Hospitals. Dr. Davenport received his medical degree from the University of Michigan, where he also did residency training in pathology and fellowship training in blood banking and transfusion medicine. Dr. Davenport's research activities have focused on the role of cytokines in hemolytic transfusion reactions, the activation of coagulation pathways by immune hemolysis, and the mechanisms of action of leukocyte-reduction filters.

Edward L. Snyder, MD, is Professor and Vice Chairman of the Department of Laboratory Medicine at Yale University School of Medicine and Director of the Blood Bank and Pheresis Service at the Yale-New Haven Hospital in New Haven, CT. Dr. Snyder was elected as the American Association of Blood Banks (AABB) President for 1997-98 and has been a member of the AABB Board of Directors for many years, serving as a Northeast District Director, Vice President, and President-Elect. He is also a member of the Editorial Board for *TRANSFUSION*.

In addition to his affiliation with the AABB, Dr. Snyder is a member of the National Institutes of Health (NIH) SBIR Study Section and has served on numerous other professional committees, including the NIH Hematology 2 Study Section, the American Society of Hematology's Transfusion Medicine Subcommittee; and the Food and Drug Administration's Blood

Products Advisory Committee. Dr. Snyder has written over 140 published abstracts and articles. His research interests include leukocyte-reduction blood filters, alterations in platelet markers during activation, storage-induced changes in platelet membrane glycoproteins and cytoskeletal proteins, platelet alloimmunization, and peripheral blood progenitor cell collection, purging, and storage.

Dr. Snyder is a graduate of the New York Medical College and completed his training at Montefiore Hospital, Bronx, NY. He is board certified in internal medicine and hematology. Dr. Snyder is a recipient of an NIH KO7 Transfusion Medicine Academic Award (TMAA) and two NIH R13 Conference Awards (1991 and 1993).

In: Davenport RD, Snyder EL, eds.
Cytokines in Transfusion Medicine: A Primer
Bethesda, MD: AABB Press, 1997

1

An Introduction to Cytokine Biology

STEVEN L. KUNKEL, PhD

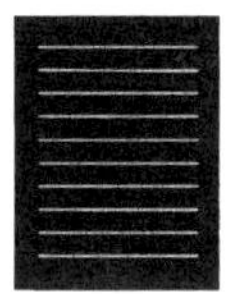

A NUMBER OF PATHOLOGIC DISEASE PROCESSES ARE dependent on a coordinated system of molecular and cellular events that participate in a complicated network of cell signaling and activation. Depending on the etiologic agent, the pathology may be limited to a restricted area of tissue injury or affect a number of systems with multiple organ involvement. It is known that a variety of chemical signals dictate the pathology associated with the progression of inflammation and tissue injury. These signals provide the basis for elaborate cell-to-cell communication cascades that are responsible for the initiation, maintenance, and resolution of a particular disorder. Several mediators are involved in the coordination of these communication networks and include: reactive nitrogen and oxygen metabolites, lipids, nucleotides, peptides, and polypeptides. This latter group of immune/inflam-

Steven L. Kunkel, PhD, Professor, Department of Pathology, The University of Michigan Medical School, Ann Arbor, Michigan

matory agents contains a large group of important mediators collectively identified as cytokines. Cytokines represent one of the largest groups of active communication signals that influence cell activation events via autocrine, paracrine, or endocrine pathways. These polypeptide mediators transmit intercellular information to specific target cells through receptor/ligand interactions and thereby regulate physiologic, immunologic, and inflammatory events.

Cytokines in Health and Disease

Cytokines may best be described as soluble polypeptides, synthesized by either immune or nonimmune cells, which dictate the controlled progression of an immune/inflammatory response. Historically, the term monokine or lymphokine was often used to denote a nonantibody protein mediator of cell immunity derived from either monocytes or lymphocytes, respectively. While the term cytokine is best used in the context of immunity and inflammation, the biologic activities of cytokines also appear to be associated with a number of normal physiologic responses.

Cytokines in Normal Physiology

Physiologists have found that certain cytokines have been implicated in normal fluctuations of body temperature, changes in slow-wave sleep, and alterations in appetite.[1-3] Interestingly, the clinical symptoms of many diseases may be due to a manifestation of elevated levels of cytokines that alter normal physiology. For example, the expression of various cytokines subsequent to an influenza infection is likely responsible for the fever, lethargy, and lack of appetite that are translated as clinical symptoms of the "flu." These exaggerated physiologic responses induced by cytokines may be an important host response to an infectious pathogen, as elevated body temperature, sleep, and reduced food intake may be key systemic components of a global host response (Fig 1-1).

Natural mediators of the pyrogenic response have long been linked to altered physiology in association with inflammation and infections. The ancient Greeks recognized the importance of a fever (calor) and classified this response as one of the four cardinal signs of the inflammatory response: calor, tumor, dolor, and rubor. Historic studies have identified that exogenous pyrogens, such as products of infectious agents or the agents themselves, can induce changes in body temperature through the production of endogenous pyrogens. The list of endogenously synthesized pyrogens is now known to consist of a variety of different cytokines with multifunctional activities.[4,5]

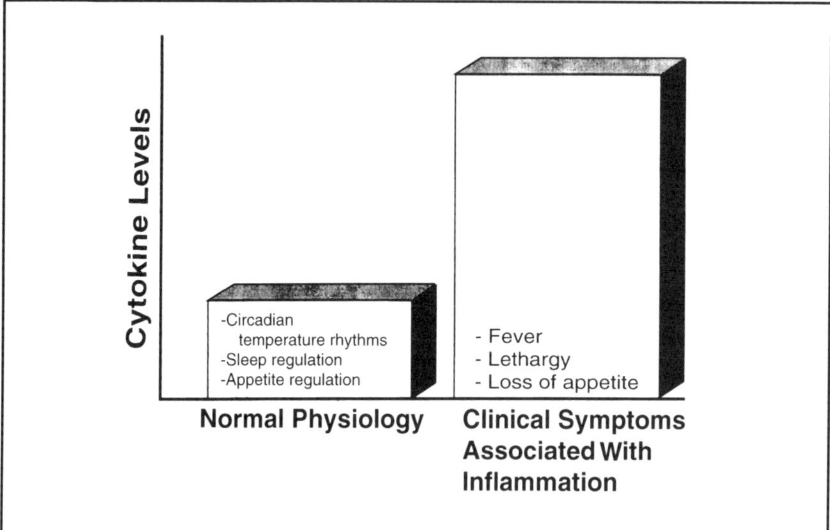

Figure 1-1. Cytokines play an important role in normal physiology; however, exaggerated physiologic responses are, in part, due to increased cytokine levels associated with the host defense response.

Of equal historical interest is the role that specific cytokines have played in dictating general metabolic responses of the host during infectious processes.[6] Cachexia, a phenomenon of general wasting and body weight loss, has been observed in patients with chronic diseases, such as tuberculosis. Interestingly, this latter disease was commonly called "consumption" because of its consuming effects on the infected host. The historic term was an accurate reflection of the grossly altered physiology associated with this chronic infectious disease, and identified the consuming, cachectic nature of excessive systemic cytokine levels.[7,8] Similar physiologic alterations are associated with other chronic disease states, including acquired immune deficiency syndrome (AIDS), cancer, and chronic granulomatous states. The actual mechanism for the altered physiology in many of these chronic diseases has not been clearly established. However, it is likely that the weight loss and cachexia associated with many chronic inflammatory diseases are associated with the over-expression of certain cytokines that alter physiology.[9]

Concentration-Dependent Effects of Cytokines

The biologic effects exhibited by cytokines in normal physiology and disease are likely concentration-dependent. During homeostasis, the concentrations of cytokines that actually interact with target cells are both low and expressed in a cyclic manner.[10] The levels that dictate specific aspects of homeostasis may actually be near the limits of detection of present cytokine assays. The concentration of cytokines that is associated with a limited immune/inflammatory response is increased over physiologic levels, but is still quite restricted. In this scenario, inflammatory cells are found in juxtaposition to one another, and tissue injury is limited. Thus, the levels of cytokines needed to facilitate limited inflammation are still low. An increase in cytokine levels can next be found in association with a more intense inflammatory response where significant leukocyte activation has occurred. Even though the inflammation may remain restricted to a given area of tissue, the levels of cytokines may reach the circulation and affect the endocrinologic system.[11] Finally, the highest levels of cytokine expression are found with systemic inflammation. In this situation, peripheral leukocytes become activated and produce high levels of cytokines, which may have a devastating effect on the host. This response can be observed during sepsis and multiorgan failure, where high levels of circulating cytokines can profoundly influence the physiology of the patient.[12-14] In these disease states, physicians often struggle to control cytokine-induced altered physiology as well as treat the etiologic agent.

Cytokine Biology

While it is clear that cytokines can induce a wide range of immunophysiologic effects in normal and disease states, there still remains the question: "To what extent do individual cytokines participate in inflammation?". As shown in Table 1-1, cytokines are an ever-growing collection of polypeptide mediators that include such diverse proteins as the interferons (IFN-α, -β, -γ), tumor necrosis factors (TNF-α, -β), colony-stimulating factors (CSFs), interleukins (IL-1 to IL-18), chemokines, and growth factors. Cytokines share a number of interesting properties that allow them to interact with cells and alter their function during an inflammatory response.

Many properties of these mediators are involved in cell activation, proliferation, phagocytosis, chemotaxis, and differentiation (Table 1-2). Thus, the biologic activities of cytokines are best described as diverse and eclectic. Cytokines are multifunctional in that the same cytokine can exert different effects in unrelated biologic systems. For example, IL-8 is both a chemotactic factor for polymorphonuclear leukocyte recruitment and an

Table 1-1. The Collection of Inflammatory Mediators Classified as Cytokines

- **Interferons** α, β, γ
  One of the first group of cytokines to be characterized.
  One of the first group of mediators with antiviral activity.
- **Tumor Necrosis Factors** α, β
  A cytotoxin in specific systems.
  Important role in cell-to-cell communication via networks.
- **Interleukins (IL-1 TO IL-17)**
  Diverse biologic activities.
  Important role in cell-to-cell communication via networks.
- **Colony-Stimulating Factors (CSFs)**
  Leukocyte colony stimulation in bone marrow.
  Leukocyte activating factor.
- **Miscellaneous Growth Factors (bFGF,PDGF, EGF)**
  Fibroblast activation factors.
  Involved in wound repair and resolution of inflammation.

angiogenic factor for the induction of neovascularization.[15,16] These are two important but quite unrelated biologic activities.

Cytokines have overlapping activities where structurally unrelated polypeptides exert the identical biologic effect during specific inflammatory events.[5] This overlapping activity can best be observed when the bio-

Table 1-2. The Activities of Cytokines on Immune/ Inflammatory Cells

- Induces cellular activation
- Promotes chemotaxis
- Promotes cell differentiation
- Augments phagocytosis
- Causes cell proliferation

logic activities of IL-1 and TNF are compared. These protein mediators are not structurally related and do not share a common receptor, yet they can induce nearly identical effects in a number of biologic systems. An additional common denominator of many cytokines is that the expression of these mediators is regulated in a complex manner, at both the transcriptional and posttranscriptional levels. This complex mechanism of cytokine regulation likely ensures that multiple steps of checks and balances are introduced into the system to control the expression of these potent compounds.

Many cytokines exhibit biphasic dose-response effects. Low concentrations can often cause a profound biologic effect, while high concentrations induce either a minimal or no effect. This latter effect may be due to the down-regulation of receptors for specific cytokines. Individual cytokines can act in a synergistic or antagonistic manner in certain biologic systems.[6] Thus, cytokines can either augment or suppress an inflammatory response.

Finally, cytokines are known to influence biologic systems through a series of cascades or networks.[17,18] The ability of cytokines to establish cell-to-cell communication is dependent on cytokine networks, in which one set of cytokines can activate immune or nonimmune cells to express an additional set of cytokines. The expression of the more distal cytokines is necessary to perpetuate and broaden the inflammatory response to include multiple participating systems. Some of the general characteristics of cytokines are found in Table 1-3, which underscores many of the complexities of these mediators.

Cytokine Classification in the Inflammatory Process

For a didactic discussion, cytokines can be categorized into four broad groups that identify their participation in various phases of the inflammatory process: activation, elicitation, removal, and resolution (Table 1-4).

The Activation and Early-Response Phase

Cytokines associated with the activation phase of the inflammatory process include early-response mediators, such as IL-1α, -β, and TNF-α.[19] These cytokines are among the first polypeptides expressed during the early phases of an inflammatory response and are key to the establishment of cytokine cascades that result in the production of other mediators. In addition to establishing cytokine networks, IL-1 and TNF are extremely important in the induction of adhesion molecules on both leukocytes and endothelial cells.[20] This is a critical early step in the evolution of an inflammatory response, as the expression of adhesion molecules on an activated or "in-

Table 1-3. The Diverse Biologic Activities of Cytokines

- **Multifunctional**
  The same cytokine can cause different effects in various systems.
- **Overlapping**
  Different cytokines can induce the same effect.
- **Biphasic Dose-Response Effects**
  A low concentration of cytokines can cause a large biologic effect.
- **Regulated in a Complex Manner**
  A variety of transcriptional and posttranscriptional factors are involved.
- **Possess Synergistic or Antagonistic Effects**
  Cytokines can augment or suppress inflammation.
- **Influence Inflammation via Cytokine Networks**
  Distal cytokines are expressed in a cascade-like manner.

Table 1-4. The Role of Cytokines in the Various Phases of Inflammation

- **Activation**
  Early response mediators, such as interleukin-1 (IL-1) and tumor necrosis factor (TNF), are key cytokines during the activation phase of inflammation.
- **Elicitation**
  Chemokines are an important group of chemotactic cytokines that are needed to deliver leukocytes successfully to an area of injury.
- **Removal**
  Cytokines, including interferon-γ (IFN-γ), are key, mediators involved in leukocyte activation for removing and killing pathogens.
- **Resolution**
  Cytokines involved in reparative processes [transforming growth factor-β (TGF-β)] are important to wound repair and healing.

flamed" endothelium serves to localize peripheral blood leukocytes to an area of tissue injury (Fig 1-2). This dynamic interaction of adhesion molecules on both circulating blood leukocytes and endothelial cells occurs in a defined sequence, which includes an initial leukocyte-rolling phenomenon followed by firm adherence of the leukocyte to the endothelium. These initial events are transient, as cell adhesion must be reversible and allow the leukocyte to leave the lumen of the vessel in order to arrive successfully at a site of tissue injury. As previously noted, these activation and early-response cytokines can also alter the host's physiology and elicit a total systemic response to the inciting agent. It is obvious that TNF and IL-1 indeed play an integral role in the evolution of an inflammatory response and have been assessed by many biotechnology and pharmaceutical companies as therapeutic targets.

The Elicitation Phase

The sequence of events that results in the recruitment of inflammatory cells from the peripheral blood to a site of tissue injury is complex. While

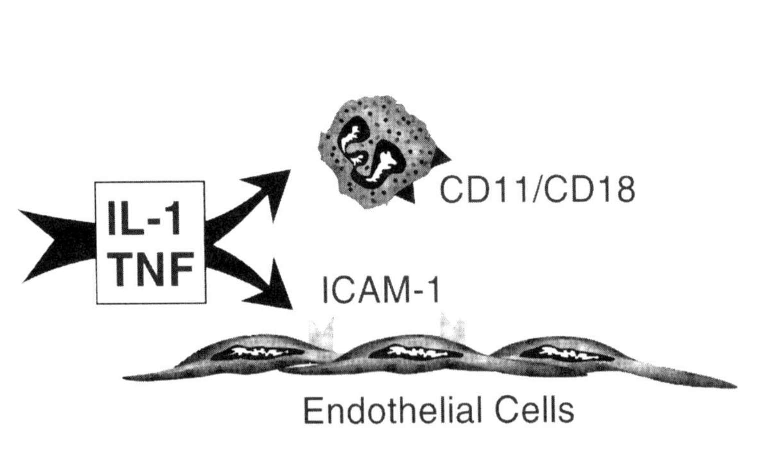

Figure 1-2. Early-response cytokines [interleukin-1 (IL-1), tumor necrosis factor (TNF)] are responsible for the rapid activation of a number of systems that promote the inflammatory response. In this example, both IL-1 and TNF are important in inducing the expression of adhesion molecules on leukocytes (CD11/CD18) and endothelial cells (ICAM-1).

the vasculature is undergoing a number of physical changes, such as vasoconstriction or vasodilatation, the inflammatory cells must adhere to the endothelium, recognize a chemotactic signal, and then undergo directed movement to an area of inflammation. The importance of leukocyte elicitation is underscored by the fact that this process can occur even during altered vessel homeostasis. The cascade of cellular events that lead to the successful elicitation of inflammatory cells is influenced by the induction and subsequent regulation of signals that modulate this dynamic recruitment process. Cytokines associated with cell elicitation are responsible for the recruitment of various subpopulations of leukocytes to a specific area of inflammation. While a high degree of redundancy can be found among chemotactic factors, the supergene family of chemokines or chemotactic cytokines is the best example of mediators that express leukocyte-recruiting activity.

Chemokines belong to specific groups of related polypeptides, which are identified by the location of two of the four cysteine amino acids that make up their primary amino acid structure.[21,22] Accumulating evidence supports the concept that members of these chemokine families have proinflammatory and reparative activities. In their monomeric form, chemokines have a molecular weight of less than 10,000 daltons and are basic heparin-binding proteins.

One of the chemokine families displays a conserved amino acid motif characterized by the location of two amino terminal cysteines separated by one nonconserved amino acid residue. This chemokine family is designated as CXC chemokines and appears to have specificity for the elicitation of mainly neutrophils. The CXC chemokines are all clustered on human chromosome 4 and possess approximately 20-55% homology in their primary structure. Interest in this area is exemplified by investigations that have identified a number of different CXC chemokines, including IL-8; platelet factor 4; platelet basic protein; connective-tissue-activating protein III; β-thromboglobulin; neutrophil-activating factor 2; growth-related oncogene-α, β, and γ; interferon gamma-inducible protein-10 (IP-10); epithelial neutrophil-activating protein-78; monokine induced by interferon gamma (MIG); and granulocyte chemotactic protein-2 (GCP-2).[23,24]

An important feature in the primary structure of CXC chemokines may account for the neutrophil chemotactic and activating properties of these mediators. Strieter et al[16] identified three critical amino acid residues immediately preceding the first N-terminal cysteine residue that are important in binding to a neutrophil receptor and activating neutrophils. These amino acids are Glu-Leu-Arg or the ELR motif, which is absent in certain members of the CXC chemokine family. In particular, IP-10, platelet factor-

4, and MIG all lack the ELR motif and are not potent in neutrophil-activating assays. Interestingly, when the ELR motif was synthetically introduced into platelet factor 4, this polypeptide gained chemotactic activity. Therefore, certain members of the CXC supergene family may have different biologic activities. Platelet factor 4 (a non-ELR-containing CXC chemokine) was one of the first members of this family to be described. This factor was originally identified for its ability to bind heparin, leading to the inactivation of the anticoagulation function of heparin.

All members of the chemokine supergene family appear to possess heparin-binding domains in their primary amino acid structure. Interleukin-8 was first identified as a monocyte-derived neutrophil chemotactic factor and has been the most studied CXC chemokine. It is produced by an array of cells, including primary cultures of monocytes, alveolar macrophages, neutrophils, keratinocytes, mesangial cells, epithelial cells, hepatocytes, fibroblasts, and endothelial cells.[25-29] In addition, IL-8 is expressed by a number of neoplasms and transformed cell lines.

Another related supergene family of polypeptide chemokines is the CC chemokine family. This group is defined by the juxtaposition of the first two N-terminal cysteines.[22] The CC chemokine family includes macrophage inflammatory protein-1 α and β; RANTES; monocyte chemoattractant protein 1, 2, and 3; I-309; and eotaxin. In general, the CC chemokine family has relative specificity for the elicitation of mononuclear cells. Certain members of the CC chemokine family also appear to be potent chemotactic factors for eosinophils. Like the CXC family, certain members of the CC family have been identified as products produced by a number of cellular sources, including lymphocytes, monocytes, neutrophils, and a variety of noninflammatory cells and tumor cell lines.

The Removal Phase

Cytokines associated with the removal phase of inflammation are those activating and differentiating factors that promote the clearance of an antigen or infectious agent. These cytokines are involved in activating either phagocytic cells (such as neutrophils, monocytes, and macrophages) or lymphocytes. One of the best studied cytokines that induce phagocytic cell activation is gamma interferon, IFN-γ.[30] This lymphocyte-derived factor is a potent stimulus for macrophage-dependent clearance of intracellular pathogens and the removal of infectious agents. IFN-γ can serve as an effective macrophage-activating factor through the induction of macrophage phagocytic activity. Such activity increases the expression of major histocompatibility complex (MHC) Class II, enhances the expression of Fc receptors on phagocytic cells, and greatly augments enzymatic activity within the cell. The activity of this cytokine also includes the induction of cytokine cascades. IFN-γ is one of the leading stimuli for the production of IL-12 by macrophages. Interleukin-12 can in turn serve as an immunoenhancing cytokine for the perpetuation of an inflammatory response.[31] While IFN-γ and IL-12 are clearly linked during leukocyte activation, leading to the removal of a specific pathogen, other cytokines are also instrumental to the successful elimination of an infectious agent. A group of cytokines that is involved with different antibody formation is fundamentally important to the removal phase of inflammation. This group includes IL-4, IL-5, IL-6, and IL-10. These different cytokines have diverse activities during immune responsiveness, but they are also involved in some phases of antibody production.

The Resolution Phase

The final phase of inflammation is characterized by wound repair and the expression of a variety of growth and angiogenic factors needed to restore normal tissue and organ function. Cytokines in this category have profound effects on fibroblast and endothelial cells and include transforming and fibroblast growth factors. These two classes of cytokines can induce fibroblast proliferation and activate fibroblasts to synthesize matrix. This latter fact is extremely important because various species of collagen are key components to end-stage reparative processes. One of the many remaining conundrums of cytokine biology is the cascade of mediators, which is active in the resolution phase of inflammation that causes either the reversible deposition of collagen or the deposition of collagen that causes permanent scarring. The former biologic response results in normal tissue restructuring and restoration of function, while the latter causes end-stage fibrosis and loss of normal tissue function.

While it is convenient to group cytokines into individual categories for didactic purposes, in reality many cytokines possess overlapping activities and appear to function in various aspects of the inflammatory response. (See Table 1-2.) Individual cytokines do possess properties that have often resulted in their historic names, such as endogenous pyrogen for IL-1 and cachectin for TNF. However, it is now known that most cytokines have multifunctional activities, which must be considered when addressing the mechanism of cytokines in the spectrum of inflammatory processes.

Proinflammatory Cytokines

The above classification of cytokines takes into account the role of cytokines in various facets of inflammation. While these categories acknowledge the complexities of cytokine biology, they do not necessarily take into account their immunopotentiating activities as key modulators of the inflammatory response. Many research laboratorians classify cytokines mainly as proinflammatory mediators because of their ability to promote inflammation (Table 1-5). These cytokines are classically involved in the initiation and maintenance of the inflammatory response and include early-response cytokines, chemotactic cytokines, and activating cytokines.

Table 1-5. A Description of Pro- and Anti-Inflammatory Cytokines

Proinflammatory Cytokines

- **IL-1 and TNF**
  Early-response cytokines are important in establishing cytokine cascades.
- **IL-8 and MCP-1**
  Chemotactic cytokines are needed to elicit blood-borne leukocytes from the lumen of a vessel to an area of inflammation.
- **IFN-γ**
  One of the most potent phagocytic cell-activating factors.
- **CSFs**
  Provide bone marrow-derived leukocytes that participate in the inflammatory response.

Anti-Inflammatory Cytokines

- **IL-10**
  Suppresses macrophage-derived cytokines, MHC Class II, and lymphocyte-derived IFN-γ.
- **IL-4**
  Regulates mononuclear phagocytic cell cytokine production.
- **TGF-β**
  Suppresses lymphocyte-derived IL-2 and blocks lymphocyte activation.

Interest in understanding these cytokines centers around the prospect of modulating inflammation by targeting these mediators for therapeutic developments. IL-1 and TNF have been prototypic proinflammatory cytokines through their multifunctional roles in dictating the evolution of an inflammatory response. This fact has not been overlooked by the pharmaceutical and biotechnology industries, as these two cytokines have been historic targets for regulation. This has been especially true with regard to the roles that IL-1 and TNF appear to play in sepsis, sepsis-like syndromes, and adult respiratory distress syndrome.[12-14] A number of Phase I and II clinical trials have been performed in an attempt to alter the production or activity of these proinflammatory mediators of inflammation. However, the fact that IL-1 and TNF are early-response cytokines and are proximal mediators of inflammation have proven to be difficult issues to overcome in designing effective therapies.

While both IL-1 and TNF are clearly proinflammatory mediators, additional cytokines are also easily classified as proinflammatory mediators. Chemokines, such as monocyte chemoattractant protein-1 and IL-8, play an intimate role in leukocyte activation and recruitment, which are fundamental processes to the initiation and maintenance of inflammation.[15] The consequences of unsuccessful leukocyte elicitation is immunosuppression; thus, this supergene family of chemotactic cytokines supports the inflammatory response in a meaningful way. Once leukocytes are successfully delivered to a site of inflammation, additional activation cytokines, including the various interferons, further perpetuate the response. As with many cytokines, interferons perform a variety of activities that cast this mediator as a central player during immune and inflammatory responses. Finally, several CSFs can also be designated as proinflammatory by providing a hemopoietic signal for the production of more leukocytes to participate in inflammation.

Anti-Inflammatory Cytokines

In addition to the growing category of proinflammatory cytokines, there is an equally extensive and important group of anti-inflammatory cytokines (Table 1-5). IL-10 is one of the best-studied members of this group. This cytokine was originally described as a Th-2-type cytokine, possessing cytokine regulatory activity.[32] Several studies have shown that IL-10 can block the expression of a number of macrophage-derived cytokines, including IL-1, TNF, IL-6, and IL-8, as well as regulate the expression of macrophage MHC Class II proteins. IL-4 and IL-13 have similar regulatory activities on macrophage-derived cytokines, as these two polypeptides can also block the expression of IL-1, TNF, and IL-8. Interestingly, these anti-inflammatory cytokines are classified as Th-2-type cytokines, are produced by T cells, and target the macrophage as a susceptible cell to regulate.

An additional group of cytokines with known immunosuppressive activities is the transforming growth factors (TGFs).[33] In particular, TGF-β is a potent suppressor of T-cell function. At low concentrations, TGF-β can block IL-2 expression, T-cell proliferation, and T-cell sensitization. The activity of TGF-β on T cells is analogous to that of IL-10, in that this latter cytokine can block T-cell cytokine production (IFN-γ) and T-cell sensitization. For the sake of discussion, it is easy to classify various cytokines as possessing one major activity. However, in reality, it is likely that various cytokines have multifunctional activities that are accentuated or suppressed depending on the global cytokine environment.

Cytokine Receptors

Investigation into how cytokines act on their target cells to elicit a specific cellular response is one of the growing areas of research into the biology of cytokines. Central to this theme is the idea that cytokines all act via cell surface receptors, resulting in an intracellular signaling response. Receptor/ligand analyses have demonstrated that many cytokines bind to their specific receptors with a high affinity, while the receptor numbers on the surface of target cells are quite low. While this latter phenomenon has hampered the purification of some cytokine receptors, several receptors have been isolated, characterized, and cloned into target cells. The use of cloned receptors expressed on target cells has provided information regarding both the molecular size of the receptor and the complex nature of a membrane-associated multimolecular receptor/ligand structure.

Cytokine Receptor Families

Recent studies have demonstrated that cytokine receptors appear to belong to specific supergene families or classes of membrane-bound proteins: the immunoglobulin-like receptor superfamily,[34] the hematopoietic receptor family,[35] and the nerve growth factor receptor family.[36] Several diverse cytokines, including IL-1, platelet-derived growth factor (PDGF), and CSF-1 bind to a cytokine receptor with structural characteristics similar to antibodies. The primary amino acid structure of the immunoglobulin-like family contains 90 conserved residues in the extracellular domain similar to those of other members of the immunoglobulin superfamily. In addition, this cytokine receptor family shares a common tertiary structure composed of two beta sheets linked by disulfide bonds.

Members of the hematopoietic receptor family also share similar amino acid structures that are found in the extracellular domain. These receptors include the binding sites for IL-2, IL-3, IL-4, IL-7, and granulocyte colony-stimulating factor (G-CSF). One of the most striking structural similarities of this family is the location of four conserved cysteine residues in one domain. It is not surprising that the similarities in the extracellular domain appear to relate directly to ligand binding; thus, many of these cytokines have a common tertiary structure that is composed of a helix bundle structure in their binding domain.

Isolation and sequencing of the cDNA for TNF receptors revealed that these two receptors are not related to those of other known cytokines, but do have structural similarities to a family of nerve growth factor receptors. The highest degree of structural homology in this family also occurs in the extracellular domain and consists of a high number of cysteine residues. The cysteine-rich regions can be further dissected into repeating regions of 80 and 40 amino acids.

While all three superfamilies of cytokine receptors possess similarities in the extracellular region, there appear to be some structural differences within the individual families. These differences are likely to confer binding specificity to the various cytokines. For example, there are additional intrachain amino acids that are different among the receptors within each class, as well as the addition and/or duplication of certain domains in individual receptors.

Soluble Receptors

A number of intriguing experiments have resulted in the identification of soluble forms of cytokine receptors.[37] In specific cases of IL-2 soluble receptor released by activated lymphocytes, the soluble nature is a result of proteolysis of the IL-2 cell surface receptor. In other cases, such as the IL-4 and IL-7 receptors, the soluble form is the product of alternative mRNA splicing instead of proteolysis of the cell surface receptor. Approximately 5-10% of the IL-4 receptor mRNA is truncated and encodes a secreted form of the intact IL-4 receptor. Specific soluble cytokine receptors have been isolated from human urine in association with various disease states. Information from these latter studies suggests that the soluble form of the cytokine receptor serves as an immunomodulating polypeptide during disease and can regulate the biologic activity of the natural cytokine ligand.

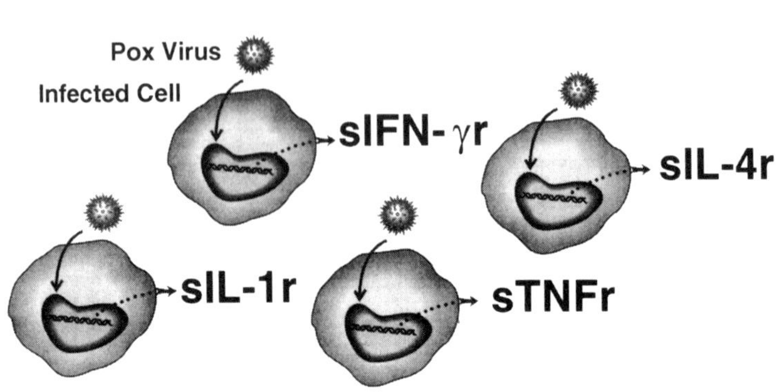

Figure 1-3. Certain DNA viruses, such as pox viruses, contain the genetic information for specific soluble cytokine receptors. Infected cells can generate significant levels of soluble receptors for INF-γ, IL-4, IL-1, and TNF. sIFN-γr = soluble gamma interferon receptor; sIL-4r = soluble IL-4 receptor; sIL-1r = soluble IL-1 receptor; sTNFr = soluble tumor necrosis factor receptor.

Virus-Directed Soluble Cytokine Receptors

Some of the best evidence for the importance of cytokines and their receptors during the evolution of an inflammatory response is derived from recent studies demonstrating that certain viruses encode soluble receptors for different cytokines (Fig 1-3). Upon expression of these cytokine receptor genes, the infected cells essentially release an immunoregulatory protein or a polypeptide that has immunosuppressive activity through its ability to bind and render reciprocal ligand cytokines biologically inactive.[38,39] The cytokines that have been targeted over the millennia of evolution by the virus are likely key host defense mechanisms that are able to mount an effective immune/inflammatory response to the viral infection. The virus has the genetic information for specific soluble cytokine receptors. When synthesized by infected cells, these polypeptides can target cytokines, such as IL-1, TNF, IL-5, and IFN-γ, and block their biologic activity. The selective removal of these key cytokines is likely to create a local environment that favors the survival of virus-infected host cells long enough for the pathogen to reach lytic maturity.

Conclusions

Investigation into the biology of cytokines has provided a number of important insights into cytokine-dependent, cell-to-cell communication networks that occur in normal physiology and disease. The activity of cytokines covers a broad range of cell-activation events that range from cell movement and activation to proliferation and differentiation. Research by both academia and industry, targeting the pro and anti-inflammatory aspects of cytokines, have provided important insights into the understanding of the biology of many cytokines. Future investigation will likely provide the information needed for the development of novel cytokine-based therapeutics for the treatment of inflammatory diseases.

References

1. Cannon JG, Kluger MJ. Endogenous pyrogen activity in human plasma after exercise. Science 1983;220:617-9.
2. Krueger JM, Walter J, Dinarello CA, et al. Sleep-promoting effects of endogenous pyrogen (interleukin-1). Am J Physiol 1984;246:R994.
3. Dinarello CA. Interleukin-1 and the pathogenesis of the acute phase response. N Eng J Med 1984;311:1413-8.
4. Davatelis G, Wolpe S, Sherry B, et al. Macrophage inflammatory protein-1: A prostaglandin-independent endogenous pyrogen. Science 1988;243:1066-8.
5. Cannon J, Tompkins RG, Geland JA, et al. Circulating interleukin-1 and tumor necrosis factor in septic shock and experimental endotoxin fever. J Infect Dis 1990;161:79-84.
6. Flores E, Bistrian B, Pomposelli J, et al. Infusion of tumor necrosis factor/cachectin promotes muscle catabolism in the rat: Synergistic effect with interleukin-1. J Clin Invest 1989;83:1614-22.
7. Old LJ. Tumor necrosis factor (TNF). Science 1985;230:630-2.
8. Beutler B, Cerami A. Tumor necrosis factor, cachexia, shock, and inflammation: A common mediator. Annu Rev Biochem 1988;57:505-18.
9. Vassalli P. The pathophysiology of tumor necrosis factors. Annu Rev Immunol 1992;10:411-52.
10. Cannon JG, Dinarello CA. Increased plasma interleukin-1 activity in women after ovulation. Science 1985;227:1247-9.
11. Oliff A, Defeo Jones D, Boyer M, et al. Tumors secreting human TNF/cachectin induce cachexia in mice. Cell 1987;50:555-63.
12. Le J, Vilcek J. TNF and IL-1: Cytokines with multiple overlapping biological activities. Lab Invest 1987;56:234-82.

13. Waage A, Halstensen A, Espevik T. Association between tumor necrosis factor in serum and fatal outcome in patients with meningococcal disease. Lancet 1987;1:355-7.
14. Girardin E, Grau GE, Dayer JM, Roux-Lombard P. Tumor necrosis factor and interleukin-1 in the serum of children with severe infectious purpura. N Engl J Med 1988;319:397-400.
15. Baggiolini M, Walz A, Kunkel SL. Neutrophil-activating peptide-1/interleukin-8, a novel cytokine that activates neutrophils. J Clin Invest 1989;84:1045-9.
16. Strieter RM, Polverini PJ, Kunkel SL, et al. The functional role of the ELR motif in CXC chemokine-mediated angiogenesis. J Biol Chem 1995;270:27348-57.
17. Standiford TJ, Kunkel SL, Basha MA, et al. Interleukin-8 gene expression by a pulmonary epithelial cell line: A model for cytokine networks in the lung. J Clin Invest 1990;86:1945-53.
18. Rolfe MW, Kunkel SL, Standiford TJ, et al. Pulmonary fibroblast expression of interleukin-8: A model for alveolar macrophage-derived cytokine networking. Am J Respir Cell Mol Biol 1991;5:493-501.
19. Beck G, Nabich GS, Benach JL, Miller F. Interleukin-1: A common endogenous mediator of inflammation and the local Schwartzman reaction. Am J Pathol 1986;125:421-32.
20. Pohlman TH, Stanness KA, Beatty PG, et al. An endothelial cell surface factor(s) induced by LPS, Il-1, and TNF alpha increases neutrophil adherences by a CDW 18-dependent mechanism. J Immunol 1986;136:45-8.
21. Matsushima K, Oppenheim JJ. Interleukin-8 and MCAF: Novel inflammatory cytokines inducible by IL-1 and TNF. Cytokine 1991;1:2-13.
22. Leonard EJ, Yoshimura T. Human monocyte chemoattractant protein-1 (MCP-1). Immunol Today 1990;11:97-100.
23. Oppenheim JJ, Zachariae OC, Mukaida N, Matsushima K. Properties of the novel proinflammatory supergene "intercrine" cytokine family. Annu Rev Immunol 1991;9:617-48.
24. Strieter RM, Standiford TJ, Rolfe MW, Kunkel SL. Interleukin-8. In: Kelley J, ed. Cytokines of the lung. New York: Marcel Dekker, Inc. 1993:281-306.
25. Rolfe MW, Kunkel SL, Standiford TJ, et al. Expression and regulation of human pulmonary fibroblast-derived monocyte chemotactic peptide-1. Am J Physiol 1992;7:536-45.
26. Strieter RM, Chensue SW, Basha MA, et al. Human alveolar macrophage gene expression of interleukin-8 by TNF-α, LPS and IL-1β. Am J Respir Cell Mol Biol 1990;2:321-6.

27. Strieter RM, Kunkel SL, Showell HJ, et al. Endothelial cell gene expression of a neutrophil chemotactic factor by TNF, LPS, and IL-1. Science 1989;243:1467-9.
28. Strieter RM, Phan SH, Showell HJ, et al. Monokine-induced neutrophil chemotactic factor gene expression in human fibroblasts. J Biol Chem 1989;264:10621-6.
29. Thornton AJ, Strieter RM, Lindley I, et al. Cytokine-induced gene expression of a neutrophil chemotactic factor-interleukin-8 by human hepatocytes. J Immunol 1990;144:2609-13.
30. Petska S, Langer JA, Zoon KC. Interferons and their actions. Annu Rev Biochem1987;56:727-45.
31. Brunda MJ. Interleukin-12. J Leuk Biol 1994;55:280-8.
32. Howard MA, O'Garra A, Ishida H, et al. Biological properties of interleukin-10. J Clin Immunol 1992;12:239-46.
33. Phan SH, Gharaee-Kermani M, McGarry B, et al. Regulation of rat pulmonary artery endothelial cell transforming growth factor-β production by IL-1β and tumor necrosis factor-α. J Immunol 1992;149:103-6.
34. Sims JE, March CJ, Cosman D, et al. cDNA expression cloning of the IL-1 receptor, a member of the immunoglobulin superfamily. Science 1988;241:585-9.
35. Nicola NA, Peterson L. Identification of distinct receptors for two hemopoeietic growth factors by chemical crosslinking. J Biol Chem 1986;261:12384-9.
36. Bazan JF. A novel family of growth factor receptors: A common binding domain in the growth hormone, prolactin, erythropoietin and IL-6 receptors, and the p75 IL-2 receptor beta chain. Biochem Biophys Res Commun 1989;164;788-95.
37. Novick D, Engelmann H, Wallach D, Rubinstein M. Soluble cytokine receptors are present in normal human urine. J Exp Med 1989;170:1409-14.
38. Smith CA, Davis T, Wignall JM, et al. T2 open reading frame from the shope fibroma virus encodes a soluble form of the TNF receptor. Biochem Biophys Res Commun 1991;176:335-42.
39. Spriggs CA, Hruby DE, Maliszewski CR, et al. Vaccina and cowpox viruses encode a novel secreted IL-1 binding protein. Cell 1992;71:145-53.

In: Davenport RD, Snyder EL, eds.
Cytokines in Transfusion Medicine: A Primer
Bethesda, MD: AABB Press, 1997

2

Cytokine Production During Blood Component Storage

GARY STACK, MD, PhD, AND
DAVID BERKOWICZ, MD, MSC

A FEBRILE, NONHEMOLYTIC, TRANSFUSION REACTION (FNHTR) is the result of immune perturbations caused by blood transfusion. The FNHTR, like fever of any origin, has autonomic, neuroimmune, and neuroendocrine components. It shares key features with the acute phase reaction to immune challenge and to the systemic inflammatory response syndrome. While a febrile response, in general, can be elicited by a host of causative agents, its manifestations are usually stereotyped. A febrile reaction to the transfusion of a blood component is typical of such a response. The stereo-

Gary Stack, MD, PhD, Chief, Pathology and Laboratory Medicine Service, VA Connecticut Healthcare System, and Assistant Professor, Department of Laboratory Medicine, Yale University School of Medicine, West Haven, Connecticut; and David Berkowicz, MD, MSC, Research Fellow, Laboratory of Computer Science, Massachusetts General Hospital, Boston, Massachusetts

typed nature of febrile responses to different pyrogenic stimuli is likely the result of a common biochemical pathway. Proinflammatory cytokines have emerged as key elements of this pathway.

Cytokines are a group of polypeptide mediators that constitute part of the soluble intercellular communication network of the immune system. They are produced by a variety of cells and play a role in coordinating and fine-tuning the immune response. Certain cytokines are now known to be pyrogenic, ie, they are capable of inducing fever. The cytokine interleukin-1 (IL-1) was the first such "endogenous pyrogen" to be identified. On the basis of our understanding of the basic mechanisms of fever generation, pyrogenic cytokines are also thought to be mediators of febrile reactions to transfusion. In the setting of a blood component transfusion, pyrogenic cytokines may be produced endogenously in transfusion recipients in response to the immune challenge of transfusion. For example, transfusion-related cytokine production in vivo may result from blood group incompatibility, leukocyte incompatibility, or bacterial contamination. Alternatively, they may be exogenously produced or secreted by donor leukocytes or platelets during component storage and be passively and inadvertently administered to recipients during transfusion. This latter mechanism is emerging as a possible leading cause of FNHTRs to platelet transfusion. The stimulus for cytokine production in the component container during storage has not been determined yet. However, it is now clear that passenger leukocytes in stored platelet concentrates remain metabolically active during blood component storage and synthesize and/or secrete cytokines and other biologic response modifiers into the plasma portion of the blood component in vitro. In addition, platelet activation or damage that occurs during the preparation and storage of platelet concentrates appears to result in the release of platelet-derived cytokines. This chapter focuses on the potential role of these "storage-generated" cytokines in FNHTRs and other nonhemolytic transfusion reactions.

The Role of Cytokines in Inflammation and Fever

Cytokine Classification

Cytokines are a diverse group of chemical-signaling molecules that can be divided into a variety of categories on the basis of their cell source or function.[1-5] The major categories include hematopoietic growth factors, interferons, lymphokines, monokines, and chemokines. This classification is somewhat arbitrary in many cases since most cytokines have multiple biologic activities and cell sources that are characteristic of more than one category. Hematopoietic growth factors are cytokines that stimulate the proliferation and differentiation of blood cells and include the colony-stimulating factors, erythropoietin, and stem cell factor. Interferons are cytokines that were originally discovered on the basis of their antiviral activity, but have other effects, including stimulation of major histocompatibility complex antigen expression and stimulation of phagocytes to attack bacteria, fungi, parasites, and tumor cells. Lymphokines are cytokines that were first described as being produced by lymphocytes, usually in response to lymphocyte stimulation, but also may be produced by other cells. Monokines are so-named because they are cytokines predominantly produced by cells of the monocyte-macrophage lineage, although they too may also be made by other cells. The monokines include IL-1, interleukin-6 (IL-6), interleukin-12 (IL-12), and tumor necrosis factor-alpha (TNF-α). Chemokines are cytokines involved in stimulating cellular chemotaxis, although they are often involved in leukocyte activation as well.[5-7]

Chemokines are further divided into two major subgroups, α and β, that are distinguished by minor structural differences on the basis of whether there is an intervening amino acid between the first two of four conserved cysteine residues. The α-chemokines all share a characteristic sequence of three amino acids at this position, two cysteines (C) separated by an intervening amino acid (X), ie, CXC. In β-chemokines, these two cysteine residues are immediately adjacent to each other, ie, CC. The α-chemokines include interleukin-8 (IL-8), β-thromboglobulin, interferon gamma-inducible protein-10 (IP-10), platelet factor 4, growth-related oncogene (GRO -α, -β, -γ); and others. The β-chemokines include macrophage inflammatory protein-1α (MIP-1α), RANTES, monocyte chemotactic protein-1, and others. Other cytokines have been characterized but they are difficult to place in the above categories because they are produced by cells other than lymphocytes or mononuclear phagocytes, their biologic action is observed mainly in concert with other cytokines, or they may both stimulate and suppress different kinds of inflammatory responses.

Inflammatory Responses and Proinflammatory Cytokines

Inflammatory reactions often consist of fever as well as leukocyte recruitment and activation at the site of immune challenge. A broader range of inflammatory responses has been classified as the acute phase response, which in addition to fever and stimulation of an immune response, encompasses changes in liver protein synthesis and/or secretion, bone marrow and endocrine changes, along with a variety of other organ and cellular responses (Fig 2-1).[4,8] In the acute phase response, the levels of some liver-derived plasma proteins, termed the acute phase proteins, increase markedly. For example, C-reactive protein and mannose-binding protein are two acute phase proteins whose increased production facilitates the removal of bacteria from the circulation as a result of their opsonizing activity. Serum amyloid protein and fibrinogen are two other acute phase proteins. In addition, energy mobilization is increased in fat and muscle cells to support the increased body temperature. Among the endocrine re-

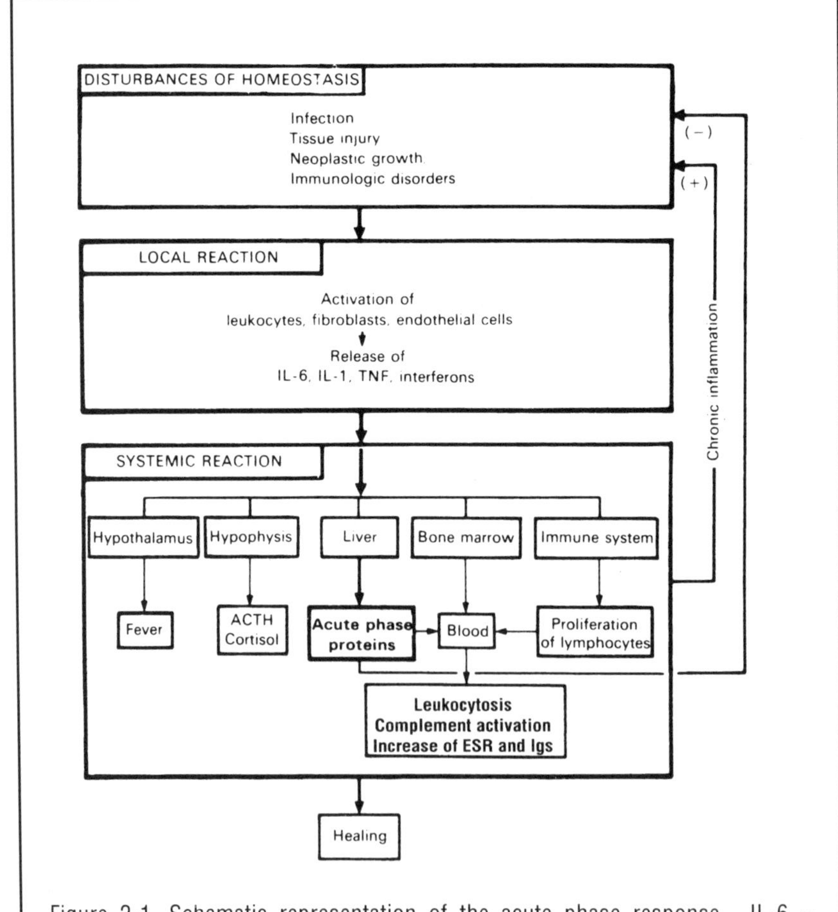

Figure 2-1. Schematic representation of the acute phase response. IL-6 = interleukin-6; IL-1 = interleukin-1; TNF = tumor necrosis factor; ACTH = adrenocorticotropic hormone; ESR = erythrocyte sedimentation rate; Igs = immunoglobulins. (Used with permission from Heinrich PC, Castell JV, Andus T.[8])

sponses, adrenocorticotropic hormone and glucocorticoids are secreted. The complement and coagulation cascades are initiated and T and B lymphocytes are activated. Leukocytes are mobilized from the bone marrow and blood vessel walls, resulting in leukocytosis. All of these responses and others provide a means by which the body attempts to restore homeostasis after an insult.

The term systemic inflammatory response syndrome (SIRS) has more recently been coined to describe some of the more easily observed or measured manifestations of the body's response to a serious insult.[9] SIRS has been commonly described in response to infection, but may be associated with noninfectious insults as well (eg, trauma, burns, ischemia, hemorrhagic shock, pancreatitis, immune-mediated organ injury, and exogenous administration of proinflammatory cytokines). It is defined as the presence of two or more of the following: body temperature higher than 38 C or lower than 36 C; heart rate more than 90 beats per minute; tachypnea (respiratory rate >20 breaths/minute, or $PaCO_2$ <32mm Hg); white blood cell count higher than 12,000/μL or lower than 4000/μL, or more than 10% immature neutrophils (band forms).[9] The SIRS criteria are clinically useful for identifying patients suffering many, if not all, of the inflammatory responses described in the acute phase response. If the acute phase response fails to restore homeostasis, SIRS may progress to the multiple organ dysfunction syndrome.[10] In such cases, the clinical consequences of the inflammatory response may be more harmful than the original insult itself.

Proinflammatory cytokines play an increasingly recognized role in mediating these inflammatory syndromes. Proinflammatory cytokines include members of several of the different cytokine subgroups described above. The first proinflammatory cytokines to be described were those with pyrogenic, ie, fever-inducing activity. Evidence for the existence of soluble mediators with pyrogenic activity was obtained by Menkin[11] and Bennett and Beeson,[12] who demonstrated that a humoral factor elaborated by white blood cells could reproduce the febrile response. Subsequent investigations have led to the isolation of a number of cytokines capable of "endogenous pyrogen" activity. The recent availability of pure recombinant protein preparations has made it possible to assess the pyrogenic activity of other cytokines. There is now good evidence that IL-1α, IL-1β, IL-6, TNF-α, the interferons, and MIP-1α act as endogenous pyrogens.[13-15] These pyrogenic cytokines alter the body's temperature regulation probably via an indirect effect on the hypothalamus (see below). Their ability to elevate body temperature may have evolved as an important component of a host's defense because many pathogens cannot grow as well at higher temperatures. In addition, adaptive immune responses may be more intense at elevated temperatures. Some proinflammatory cytokines have additional biologic activities that help coordinate the body's responses to infection and other immune challenges.[4] Some increase energy mobilization through their actions on muscle and fat cells. IL-1 and IL-6 also contribute to the adaptive immune response by helping to activate B and T cells, and IL-6 is a major regulator of acute phase protein synthesis. The chemokines, such as IL-8, MIP-1α, and many others, play a role in the inflammatory response as chemotactic factors that recruit leukocytes to sites of infection or immune challenge, and in some cases also activate leukocytes.[5-7]

The Role of Cytokines in the Pathogenesis of Fever

The mechanism for the increase in body temperature in fever, in general, and presumably in FNHTRs, appears to be a cytokine-mediated up regulation of the thermostatic set point for body temperature in the preoptic area of the anterior hypothalamus (Fig 2-2).[14-20] Circulating pyrogenic cytokines, such as IL-1β, IL-6, and TNF-α, appear to achieve thermoregulatory effects by first stimulating prostaglandin (PG) E_2 production in the anterior hypothalamus. The production of prostaglandins appears to be an important step in the pathogenesis of fever since it is known that PG inhibitors such as aspirin and indomethacin block the generation of fever. Cyclooxygenase, a key enzyme involved in the synthesis of PG, is, in fact, found in the central nervous system in microglia, astrocytes, and neurons. The PGs in turn presumably reach the thermosensitive neurons in the preoptic area of the anterior hypothalamus by diffusion. This area of the brain appears to be involved in temperature regulation through the coordinated firing of "hot-" and "cold-" sensitive neurons. Fever is associated with a decrease in the firing rate of the "warm" neurons and an increase in the firing of the "cold" neurons.[14,18] However, some fevers appear to be mediated by mechanisms that do not involve prostaglandins. Perhaps, in some cases, alterations in firing rates of thermosensitive neurons occur via direct cell-to-cell contacts with cytokine-responsive neurons. This might explain why fever induced by MIP-1α is not prevented by ibuprofen.[21]

Chills and rigors are part of the mechanism by which body temperature is elevated and frequently precede the onset of fever. Rigors, or shaking chills, are the result of muscle contractions that increase heat generation. The sensation of a chill may be due at least in part to a peripheral vasoconstriction that shunts blood centrally for heat conservation. Behavioral changes also may contribute to increased body temperature. For example, an affected individual may cover up for increased warmth to cope with a perceived chill.

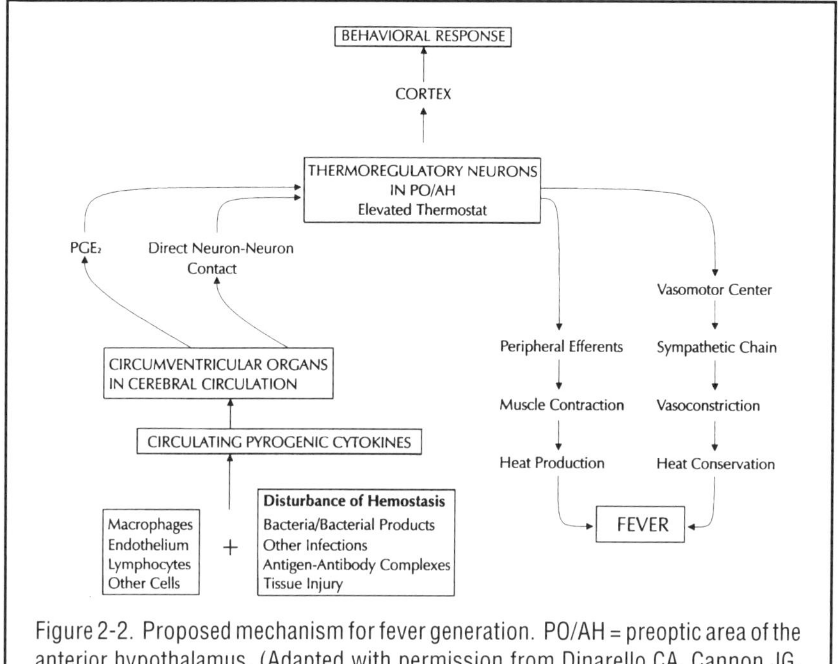

Figure 2-2. Proposed mechanism for fever generation. PO/AH = preoptic area of the anterior hypothalamus. (Adapted with permission from Dinarello CA, Cannon JG, Wolff SM.[16])

It is not clear whether or how pyrogenic cytokines reach the thermoregulatory regions of the brain, since these regions are not in ready contact with the bloodstream because of the blood-brain barrier.[14,15,19] This has raised questions regarding whether intravascular levels of cytokines are even involved in fever generation. A number of possible mechanisms discussed later in this chapter have been proposed to account for the ability of circulating pyrogens to breach this barrier and cause their central effects.

Cytokines and Febrile Nonhemolytic Transfusion Reactions

The Role of Inflammatory Syndromes in Transfusion Reactions

Serious transfusion reactions caused by immune-mediated acute hemolysis or the infusion of bacterially contaminated blood components represent major immunologic insults that may provoke the full extent of the SIRS and many aspects of the acute phase response. On the other hand, most FNHTRs (see below) are probably mild versions of these inflammatory syndromes and seem at least outwardly to be largely confined to changes in vital signs, eg, body temperature and respiratory rate. Some of the most serious FNHTRs will meet the minimum criteria of SIRS. Because proinflammatory cytokines mediate fever and play a major role in inducing the inflammatory syndromes, we expect that they will likewise play a major role as mediators of FNHTRs.

Description of a Febrile Nonhemolytic Transfusion Reaction

A febrile reaction to transfusion is classified as a febrile, nonhemolytic, transfusion reaction if no other identifiable cause of fever exists and laboratory investigations reveal no evidence of hemolysis of transfused red blood cells or bacterial contamination of the blood component.[22,23] FNHTRs often start with the patient experiencing chills. In some cases, a patient may suffer a mild reaction by experiencing chills with no fever. A fever may develop between a half-hour to several hours after the start of the transfusion. The symptoms of FNHTRs are usually self-limited and the fever does not usually last more than 8-12 hours after transfusion. Fevers persisting 18-24 hours or more are unlikely to be transfusion-related. Higher rates of temperature elevation after transfusion can be associated with faster rates of infusion and/or a greater passenger leukocyte content of the blood component.[24] The incidence of FNHTRs has been estimated at 0.5% per unit of blood component transfused; however, substantial variability in reaction rates has been reported.[25,26] Reactions to transfusions of multiunit pools of platelet concentrates have been reported to be as high as 20-30% at some centers.[22] Pools of platelet concentrates (PCs) from several donors, in fact, have been reported to cause a higher rate of FNHTRs than single-donor apheresis platelets.[27] Reactions are also more frequent in certain recipients, namely, those patients who have been previously exposed to multiple white cell and platelet antigens.[28] This group includes multiparous women and multitransfused patients.

Evidence That Soluble Mediators Induce FNHTRs

It has been widely held that most FNHTRs are mediated by recipient leukocyte antibodies that bind to infused passenger leukocytes from the transfused blood component. The resulting immune complex formation may directly activate lymphocytes or monocytes to produce pyrogenic cytokines or result in complement activation that in turn stimulates pyrogenic cytokine generation by mononuclear cells. This mechanism is consistent with observations made over several decades of study of FNHTRs to red blood cell (RBC) transfusion and remains the leading explanation for

FNHTRs to the transfusion of RBCs.[24,29-35] However, this etiology is inconsistent with more recent observations involving FNHTRs to platelet transfusions.

For example, Chambers et al[27] noted that a significant number of FNHTRs are observed in individuals receiving platelet transfusion for the first time and who have not been previously pregnant. It is unlikely that these reactions could have been mediated by recipient leukocyte antibodies since the recipients had no prior exposure to foreign leukocytes. Furthermore, leukocyte reduction by bedside filtration has given disappointing results in reducing FNHTRs to platelet transfusion. In fact, on the basis of published studies and anecdotal reports, it is unclear whether bedside leukocyte reduction has any significant effect on the rate of FNHTRs to platelets. For example, Mangano et al[36] observed a higher rate of FNHTRs to bedside leukocyte-reduced platelet concentrates than would have been predicted from the degree of leukocyte reduction. In addition, Goodnough et al[37] actually observed a statistically significant increase in FNHTRs in a population of oncology patients receiving bedside, leukocyte-reduced platelets when compared with historic controls. These results suggest that some element other than the leukocyte content of platelet preparations at the time of transfusion may mediate FNHTRs. Moreover, Muylle et al[38] and Heddle et al[39] have observed that the rate of FNHTRs to older units of PCs is higher than to fresher units, suggesting that a storage-related change contributes to the reactions. Finally, Heddle et al[40] reported that the plasma portion of PCs causes a higher rate of chill reactions than the cellular portion containing the passenger leukocytes. They divided pools of PCs into cellular and plasma portions and transfused each portion separately into the same recipient in random order with a 2-hour interval between infusions. Their results indicate that chill reactions are induced in most cases by the plasma portion of PCs and not by the cellular portion containing the leukocytes and platelets. Taken together these results suggest that a soluble, rather than a cell-associated, factor is involved in mediating many FNHTRs occurring in response to platelet transfusions, and that this soluble factor increases during PC storage.

The Generation of Cytokines in Stored Platelet Concentrates

Several groups have demonstrated that a variety of pyrogenic or other proinflammatory cytokines, such as IL-1β, IL-6, IL-8, TNF-α, MIP-1α, GRO-α, RANTES, and transforming growth factor-β (TGF-β), can be measured in the plasma portion of stored PCs.[40-51] Because of their biologic activities, many of these are plausible candidates to be mediators of FNHTRs, if infused in sufficiently high amounts. Moreover, they meet the criteria described above of being present in the plasma/supernatant portion of platelet concentrates and of having increased concentrations in older units of PCs (see below).

Stack and Snyder[41,43] showed that significant amounts of IL-8, IL-1β, IL-6, and TNF-α accumulate over time in the plasma portion of PCs during routine blood bank storage. They reported a mean IL-8 concentration of 11,600 pg/mL and a maximal level of 212,000 pg/mL in 5-day-old PCs. IL-1β, IL-6, and TNF-α were detected in units that contained relatively high levels of IL-8, but at significantly lower concentrations (see Table 2-1). The percentage of platelet concentrates with detectable IL-8 ranged from 30% in 2-day-old units to 83% in 5-day-old units. Muylle et al[42] also detected IL-1β, IL-6, and TNF-α in stored PCs, but at higher levels than those measured by Stack and Snyder.[43] They detected mean levels of IL-1β and IL-6 of about 5000 pg/mL and a mean level of TNF-α of about 600 pg/mL by 5 days of storage. These higher levels may reflect their use of protease inhibitors to prevent proteolytic degradation of cytokines following sampling. The higher levels may also be related to the approximate two-and-a-half-fold higher leukocyte content of the PCs they studied. Heddle et al[40] also detected IL-1β and IL-6 in stored PCs. They found relatively low levels of IL-1β (median = 14 pg/mL), but comparatively higher levels of IL-6 (median = 540 pg/mL) in 5-day-old PCs. Unlike the other investigators, Heddle et al[40] used a bioassay rather than an enzyme immunoassay for IL-6, which might explain some differences in the results of other studies. Aye et al[44] reported values of IL-1β, IL-6, IL-8, and TNF-α similar to those of Stack and Snyder,[42] with IL-8 being present at the highest level (mean = 7600 pg/mL). With the exception of the study of Muylle et al,[42] TNF-α has been measured at only very low levels (<100 pg/mL).

It is frequently difficult to make a direct and meaningful comparison between reports from different centers because they have a number of uncontrolled variables, such as different methods of platelet preparation, differences in the leukocyte content of units of PCs, differences in sampling technique, and different assays. For example, PCs prepared from buffy coats appear to contain little, if any, cytokines in their plasma portion compared with PCs prepared from platelet-rich plasma.[52,53] This may be largely explained by their lower passenger leukocyte content. Moreover, apheresis platelets also appear to contain lower levels of some plasma cytokines, such as IL-8, perhaps again related to their lower leukocyte content made possible with current apheresis instrumentation.[54] Despite the variation in the cytokine concentrations reported, the developing consensus of the relative

Table 2-1. Leukocyte-Derived Cytokines in Platelet Concentrates at Storage Day 5*

	Muylle et al[42]		Stack and Snyder[43]		Heddle et al[40]		Aye et al[44]	
Cytokine	**Mean**	**Max**	**Mean**	**Max**	**Median**	**Max**	**Mean**	**Max**
IL-1β	5250	26,000	—	>2000	14	143	105	—
IL-6	4883	17,000	—	737	540	10,000	269	—
IL-8	—	—	11,600	212,000	—	—	7600	—
TNF-α	571	1890	—	55	—	—	42	—

*Data are expressed as pg/mL. IL = interleukin; TNF = tumor necrosis-α; IL-1β = interleukin-1β.

quantities of storage-generated, leukocyte-derived cytokines in PCs derived from platelet-rich plasma is: IL-8 >> IL-1β > IL-6 > TNF-α.

More recently, platelet-derived cytokines have also been investigated. Several additional members of the chemokine family of cytokines, including RANTES, platelet factor 4, β-thromboglobulin, GRO-α, and MIP-1α, have been detected in the supernatant portions of PCs.[45-49,55] These chemokines are apparently stored in the α granules of platelets, although GRO-α and MIP-1α may also be leukocyte-derived.[49] Transforming growth factor-β, a platelet-derived cytokine that is not a chemokine, has also been detected in the plasma portion of PCs.[47] Unlike leukocyte-derived cytokines, platelet-derived cytokines with the exception of GRO-α and MIP-1α are generally present at higher concentrations and accumulate earlier in storage.

Factors Affecting Cytokine Levels in Platelet Concentrates

Leukocyte Content

The accumulation of leukocyte-derived cytokines, such as IL-1β, IL-6, IL-8, and TNF-α appears to be proportional to the passenger leukocyte content of many platelet concentrates. Stack and Snyder[41,43] correlated a high plasma concentration of leukocyte-derived cytokines with a high passenger leukocyte count (Fig 2-3). Conversely, a low level of cytokines correlated with a low leukocyte count. Nearly all (ie, 97%) of the units of PCs with IL-8 levels greater than 1000 pg/mL had either a WBC greater than 2000/μL or a storage time of at least 4 days. On the other hand, they did not detect significant levels of IL-8, IL-1β, IL-6, or TNF-α in units with a WBC of less than 1000/μL and a storage time of less than 4 days. Muylle et al[42] observed a similar dependence of cytokine production on passenger leukocyte content, but in their case saw no cytokine accumulation up to 5 days of storage when the passenger leukocyte content was less than 3000/μL. The dependence of cytokine production on passenger leukocyte content is further demonstrated by the effect of prestorage leukocyte reduction. Prestorage white cell reduction using third-generation filters that are expected to reduce the leukocyte count by about three logs was shown to prevent the accumulation of IL-1β, IL-6, IL-8, and TNF-α up to day 5 of storage.[40,43,44,56]

Storage Time

Levels of leukocyte-derived cytokines in the plasma portion of PCs at day 0 or 1 of storage have been found to be very low or nondetectable. Stack and

Snyder[41,43] did not detect any IL-1β or IL-8 on day 1 of storage in 17 units of PCs tested. Similar results were reported by others, although in some studies low levels of leukocyte-derived cytokines, usually near the limit of detection, were detected on day 0 or 1 of storage.[40,42,44] The mean levels of plasma cytokines were shown to increase with increasing storage times up to 5 days (Fig 2-3).[40-44] Aye et al[44] determined that there was a significant increase in the levels of IL-1β, IL-6, IL-8, and TNF-α from day 0 to day 3, followed by a nonsignificant "increment" from day 3 to day 5. Overall, the evidence suggests that these leukocyte-derived cytokines are generated and accumulate in PCs during routine blood bank storage and are not released in significant amounts during blood donation or component preparation. Units with longer storage times can be expected to have higher cytokine levels. However, it must be kept in mind that units with a low leukocyte content will generally not have detectable leukocyte-derived cytokines even after 5 days of storage.

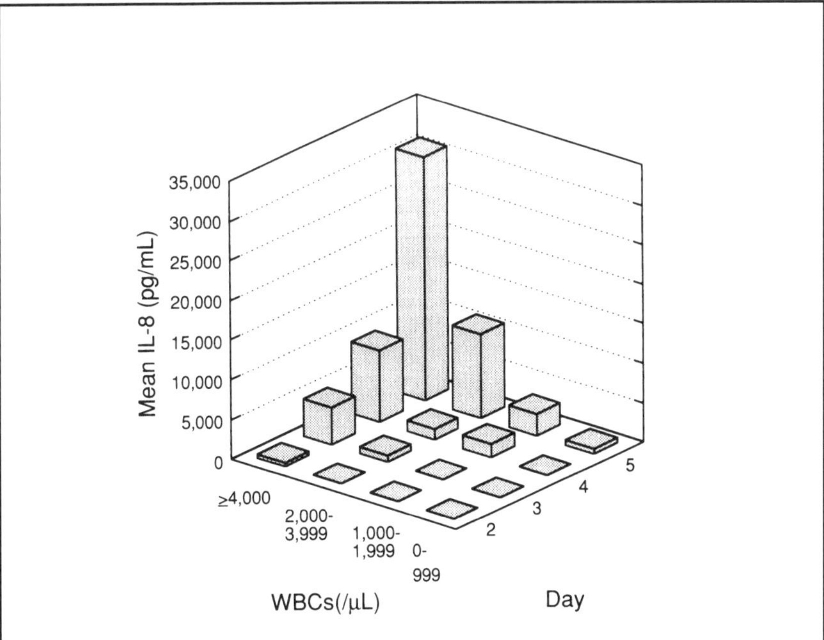

Figure 2-3. IL-8 levels in platelet concentrates in relation to WBC count and storage time. The ordinate represents the mean IL-8 levels in platelet concentrates with the indicated WBC content (cells/μL) and storage time (days). IL-8 = interleukin-8; WBCs = white blood cells. (Used with permission from Stack G, Snyder EL.[44])

Storage Temperature

PCs are stored at room temperature (20-24 C), which could be expected to allow cytokine-producing mononuclear cells to sustain some metabolic activity. Stack et al[57] measured levels of IL-1β and IL-8 in the supernatant portion of units of additive solution RBCs stored at 1-6 C and found the cytokine accumulation to be significantly lower over 42 days than in PCs stored at room temperature over 5 days. This result suggests that the colder storage temperature of RBCs may have an inhibitory effect on cytokine accumulation. However, numerous other differences in storage conditions of RBC units and PCs could also account for this result. To address this issue further, Heddle et al[58] directly compared cytokine accumulation in PCs stored in the cold with those stored at room temperature and indeed found that cold storage inhibited cytokine accumulation in the plasma portion of PCs. These data indicate that storage of PCs and likely other blood components in the cold is one way of preventing cytokine accumulation. These data are consistent with the concept that cytokine generation occurs by an active, temperature-dependent, metabolic process.

Bacterial Contamination

Based on studies of the inflammatory response syndrome that accompanies sepsis, proinflammatory cytokines are known to be stimulated in vivo in response to some bacteria and bacterial products.[59-62] For this reason, proinflammatory cytokines likely play a major role in the symptom complex of septic transfusion reactions that occur when transfusion recipients are infused with bacterially contaminated blood components. Moreover, some uncomplicated FNHTRs may also result from the transfusion of blood components with low levels of bacterial contamination. Bacterial contamination of a donor unit may result from inadequate preparation of the donor's arm, leading to the introduction of skin flora into the donated blood, or from an undetected donor bacteremia. The potential sources of cytokines in the setting of septic transfusion include: 1) recipient leukocytes and other cell types activated in response to bacterial infusion, 2) donor leukocytes after infusion, and 3) donor leukocytes in the blood component container exposed to bacteria or their products in vitro. It seems likely that recipient leukocytes and other cells would be the major source of cytokines in septic transfusion reactions. However, this does not preclude a physiologic role of cytokines produced in vitro by stimulated donor leukocytes.

Bacteria in stored units of PCs, and to a lesser extent in units of RBCs, provoke further increases in the levels of plasma cytokines in vitro.[57,63] Inoculation of PCs on day 1 or day 2 of storage with *Escherichia coli*, a gram-negative, endotoxin-producing organism, has been shown to stimulate IL-8 levels in the supernatant fluid from 6- to 16-fold.[63] Similarly, the concentrations of IL-1β and another chemokine, MIP-1α, were likewise increased. In addition, contamination with *Yersinia enterocolitica* stimulates IL-1β and IL-8 in units of additive-solution RBCs progressively over 42 days of storage.[57] While this effect of bacterial contamination is statistically significant in units of RBCs, the average stimulation is less than two-fold. Maximal levels of cytokines in RBC units after contamination with *Y. enterocolitica* or *Staphylococcus aureus* were typically lower than 30 pg/mL for IL-1β and lower than 3000 pg/mL for IL-8. While the increased levels of cytokines in bacterially contaminated PCs could theoretically play a role in the early manifestations of septic reactions, the significance of the lower levels in units of RBCs is less clear.

Other Factors

It is likely that other variables also determine the levels of cytokines that accumulate in stored PCs. In some cases, units of PCs may have similar leukocyte contents and storage times, yet have markedly different plasma cytokine levels. The explanation for this is unknown, but may possibly be related to variations in the presence of inciting stimuli, whatever they may be, from unit to unit. The responsiveness of passenger leukocytes to cytokine-producing stimuli may also vary between units of PCs. For example, differences in responsiveness in vitro may be related to differences in the donors' immune responsiveness. Such differences are known to exist, such as the greater immune responsiveness of females, in general, compared with that of males. In fact, steroid sex hormones have been shown to regulate macrophage release of tumor necrosis factor.[64] It is possible that other variables may also affect cytokine generation, such as the type of plastic or plasticizer in the container wall. Adherence to plastic is a known stimulus for monocytes to synthesize and secrete cytokines (see below), and differences in plastics used in container manufacture might be of significance. Other treatments or manipulations of blood components, such as gamma and ultraviolet irradiation, may also modulate cytokine accumulation. Preliminary data reveal a minimal effect of low-dose gamma irradiation.[65] On the other hand, high-dose ultraviolet irradiation appears to have an inhibitory effect.[65] Confirmation of these results, however, is necessary.

The Generation of Cytokines During the Storage of Red Blood Cells

While cytokine accumulation has been most extensively studied in PCs, proinflammatory cytokines have also been measured in the supernatant portions of units of additive solution RBCs.[57,66] Unlike platelet concentrates, which are stored at 20-24 C for up to 5 days, additive solution RBCs are stored at 1-6 C for up to 42 days. The cold temperature would be expected to inhibit the metabolism of passenger leukocytes in units of RBCs and thereby inhibit the synthesis of cytokines during storage. On the other hand, release of preexisting intracellular stores of cytokines during cell lysis might be as great or greater in units of RBCs than in PCs because of their longer storage time. Studies by Stack et al[57] and Smith et al[66] revealed the presence of IL-8 and, to a lesser extent, IL-1β in the supernatant portion of units of additive solution-1 (AS-1) RBCs. Levels of IL-8 and IL-1β increased progressively, but slowly, over 42 days of storage. IL-8 levels ranged from about 200-2000 pg/mL by 42 days of storage, whereas IL-1β levels never exceeded 13 pg/mL.[57] IL-6 was not detected in any unit tested. Because of the much lower level of plasma cytokines generated in RBC units compared with PCs, storage-generated, proinflammatory cytokines in RBC units appear to be less likely to have physiologic significance. However, some effect has not been ruled out. For example, IL-8 may have a priming effect on passenger leukocytes that renders them more sensitive to other cytokines they might encounter in vivo after transfusion into the recipient.[67] Moreoever, low levels of some cytokines are known to act synergistically with other cytokines.[68-70]

Sources and Stimulus for Cytokine Accumulation in Stored Blood Components

The source of the proinflammatory cytokines IL-1β, IL-6, IL-8, and TNF-α in stored PCs and RBCs is presumably the passenger leukocytes. Platelets are not known to be large reservoirs of these typically leukocyte-derived cytokines and red blood cells are not known to contain these cytokines. Moreover, as discussed above, the accumulation of these cytokines is proportional to the leukocyte content of the units. In addition, the removal of leukocytes early in storage prevents the accumulation of IL-1β, IL-6, IL-8, and TNF-α during subsequent storage. Monocytes are a likely source of these cytokines, although other leukocytes have not been ruled out.

The accumulation of cytokines in the plasma supernatant portion of units of PCs and RBCs could be the result of 1) new synthesis and secretion, 2) secretion of preexisting cellular stores, or 3) release of cellular contents during cell degradation. Muylle et al[42] attempted to determine if new synthesis accounted for the increases they observed during storage by measuring total intra- and extracellular levels of IL-1β, IL-6, and TNF-α in cell lysates of samples taken from PCs over 7 days of storage. Total bag contents of all three cytokines increased over 7 days of storage, ranging from a 30-fold increase in TNF-α to about an 800-fold increase in IL-6. Thus, the accumulation of these cytokines was apparently the result of new polypeptide synthesis and not solely the result of secretion or degradative release of preexisting stores. Takahashi et al[65] measured IL-8 messenger (mRNA) levels at varying storage times in apheresis platelets. Their results showed an increase in IL-8 mRNA with increasing storage time, indicating that the increase in IL-8 could be due at least in part to new synthesis resulting from increased gene transcription or mRNA stability.

The stimulus or stimuli for cytokine generation in stored cellular blood components is not yet known. Since cytokine accumulation occurs in individual, unpooled units of PCs or RBCs, an immunologic incompatibility is not the inciting stimulus. However, other stimuli are potentially present (see Table 2-2). For example, monocytes among the passenger leukocytes might undergo contact activation on interaction with the plastic wall of the blood component bag. Adherence to plastic surfaces has been reported to stimulate the production of cytokines by monocytes in cell culture.[71-73] In support of this hypothesis, Elkattan et al[74] reported a correlation between the adherence of mononuclear cells to plastic bag walls and cytokine levels in units of apheresis platelets. Monocytes in blood components may also be

Table 2-2. Potential Stimuli for Cytokine Release From Monocytes in Platelet Concentrates

- Contact activation due to adherence to plastic container wall
- Adherence to activated platelets
- Complement activation
- Bacterial products
- Microdamage
- Plasticizer
- Apoptosis
- Hypoxia

induced to secrete cytokines by interaction with activated platelets. Platelets progressively undergo activation during platelet storage until 40-60% are in an activated state by day 5 of storage.[75] During the process of activation, platelets translocate the adhesion molecule P-selectin to their surface from intracellular storage granules. P-selectin on the surface of platelets binds to P-selectin glycoprotein ligand-1 on the surface of monocytes to mediate platelet-monocyte adhesion. This adhesion to activated platelets has been shown to signal monocytes to synthesize and secrete cytokines, including the chemokines IL-8 and monocyte chemotactic protein-1.[76]

Table 2-2 lists a variety of additional potential stimuli. Complement activation, for example, occurs during PC storage and monocytes are known to be activated to produce cytokines in cell culture by activated complement components.[77-79] Endotoxin or other bacterial products also may be present in at least some bags at a level sufficient to induce monocytes to produce cytokines. This is almost certainly the case in bacterially contaminated units. Endotoxin is a known potent stimulus for inflammatory cytokines in sepsis, and cytokine production by monocytes in culture was shown to be exquisitely sensitive to low concentrations of endotoxin.[59,62,80] To show that this mechanism is possible, Stack and coworkers[57,63] observed increases in IL-1β, IL-8, and MIP-1α in units of PCs experimentally contaminated with *E. coli*, as well as increases in IL-1β and IL-8 in units of RBCs inoculated with *Y. enterocolitica*. Plasticizers used in the manufacture of blood component containers are another potential stimulus. The plasticizer diethylhexylphthalate, commonly used as a plasticizer in primary blood collection bags and in some platelet containers, has been shown to stimulate IL-1 secretion by monocytes in short-term culture.[81] The relative hypoxia of monocytes during component preparation and blood bank storage is another possible contributor to cytokine release, since mononuclear and endothelial cells subjected transiently to anoxic conditions in culture have been shown to secrete IL-8.[82,83] Monocyte injury, which may occur at various stages of blood component preparation and storage, has also been shown to cause cytokine release. For example, "microdamage" to monocyte cell membranes can cause an unregulated release of IL-1β.[84] Moreover, in monocyte apoptosis, or regulated cell death, IL-1β is processed and released in its mature form.[85] It is possible, although untested, that PC storage conditions induce monocyte damage or apoptosis, thereby leading to cytokine release. The stimulus for the release of platelet-derived cytokines during platelet storage, as with leukocyte-derived cytokines, has not been determined, but could be related to platelet activation or damage.

The cytokines released during blood component storage possibly have feedback on each other's synthesis or secretion. From cell culture studies the interrelationships of various proinflammatory cytokines appear complex. For example, IL-1β can stimulate the production of TNF-α and vice versa.[80,86] TNF-α and IL-1β stimulate the production of IL-6 and IL-8.[7,87,88] In addition, TGF-β and IL-6 can suppress the production of IL-1.[80,89,90] Thus, the generation of some cytokines could possibly be the result of the sequential action of other cytokines. Further work is necessary to determine what role these or other stimuli have in the generation of cytokines in stored PCs and RBCs.

Effects of Prestorage Leukocyte Reduction

Several laboratories have shown that early or prestorage leukocyte reduction by filtration prevents or substantially reduces cytokine accumulation in units of both PCs and RBCs during subsequent blood bank storage. Stack and Snyder[43] observed a dramatic reduction in the IL-8 levels at 5 days of storage to below the level of detection (ie, <18 .1 pg/mL) in early-storage, leukocyte-reduced PCs. They observed a similar elimination of IL-1β. Muylle and Peetermans[56] observed that leukocyte reduction within 12 hours of platelet preparation eliminated IL-1β, IL-6, and TNF-α accumulation during subsequent storage. Heddle et al[40] also observed the elimination of IL-1β and the reduction of IL-6 levels to near zero with early-storage leukocyte reduction by filtration. Aye et al[44] confirmed the earlier observation of these groups by showing that leukocyte reduction prevents the accumulation of IL-8, IL-1β, IL-6, and TNF-α in stored PCs. Stack et al,[57] measuring cytokines in units of RBCs, observed that the relatively low levels of IL-8 and IL-6 that accumulated over 42 days of storage also could be substantially reduced by early-storage (day 3) leukocyte reduction of the units. Stack et al[57,63] also demonstrated that early-storage leukocyte reduction by filtration prior to bacterial contamination effectively prevented any stimulatory effect of bacterial contamination on levels of IL-1β and IL-8 in both PCs and RBCs. Thus, prestorage leukocyte reduction appears to be an effective way to prevent or reduce leukocyte-derived cytokine accumulation.

The Physiologic Significance of Storage-Generated Cytokines

Are Cytokine Levels in PCs High Enough to Cause Reactions?

The key to whether storage-generated cytokines potentially mediate adverse responses in transfusion recipients is whether the cytokine content of the blood components is sufficiently high to be of physiologic significance. Insight into this comes from toxicity studies of purified recombinant cytokines given intravenously to human recipients. The administration of intravenous IL-1β in humans at doses ranging from 10-100 ng/kg has produced fever, headaches, myalgias, arthralgias, and gastrointestinal symptoms.[80] Lower doses of 1-10 ng/kg have also produced fever, rigors, and transient tachycardia.[91,92] On the basis of these studies, it can be concluded that intravenous doses of from 70-7000 ng of IL-1β in a 70-kg individual are capable of inducing fever, chills, and other symptoms. Using published cytokine levels in PCs (see Table 2-1), the calculated mean IL-1β content in a 300/mL, 6-unit pool of PCs ranges from 4-1600 ng, depending on the study. Thus, the plasma levels of IL-1β in some PCs is within the dose range capable of causing febrile reactions. Of course, one would not expect that all pools of PCs should have a physiologically significant dose because not all transfusions result in fever.

The intravenous administration of recombinant human TNF-α has been reported to cause rigors at a dose of 5 μg/m^2 in one study[93] and fever at a dose of 10 μg/m^2 in another.[94] Thus, in an individual with a body surface area of 1.7 m^2, total doses in the range of 8500-17,000 ng would cause rigors and fever. By comparison of published studies (see Table 2-1), the mean content of TNF-α in a 300 mL pool of PCs ranges from 13-171 ng. If all units in the pool had the highest known level of TNF-α, the total estimated content would be between 17 and 567 ng. Thus, it is unclear whether the dose of TNF-α present in PCs is capable of inducing fever. However, there is an increased chance that the infused TNF-α would approach physiologic significance in a transfusion recipient of smaller body mass, such as small adults or children. Also, at this time, one cannot rule out the possibility that TNF-α in PCs may have an additive or synergistic effect with other cytokines.

Mean IL-8 levels reported in the plasma portion of PCs were 7600 pg/mL and 11,600 pg/mL in two studies.[43,44] Levels as high as about 200 ng/mL have been detected in some PCs.[43] On the basis of these values, the mean total IL-8 content in a pool of six units of PCs is expected to be between 200 ng to 3500 ng. The content could be as high as 13 μg if one unit with 200 ng/mL were pooled with five other units with the mean observed level. The mean plasma level of IL-8 associated with SIRS in endotoxin-injected human volunteers in one study was 641 pg/mL.[62] Assuming a 3000/mL plasma volume, the total intravascular content of IL-8 in that setting is 1923 ng. This level appears achievable from a transfusion source even if substantial extravascular partitioning of IL-8 occurs in vivo.

IL-8 itself appears not to induce fever in humans and so might be considered an unlikely candidate to mediate FNHTRs. However, it does prime leukocytes to increase their sensitivity to other cytokines that are pyrogenic, such as TNF-α.[67] In that way, IL-8 might still contribute to FNHTRs. IL-8 stimulates neutrophil chemotaxis, activation, and degranulation, as well as basophil release of histamine.[5-7,95,96] Plasma levels of IL-8 in sepsis are correlated with the severity of sepsis syndrome.[87,97] Intravenous infusions of IL-8 in nonhuman primates cause transient granulocytopenia followed by a rebound granulocytosis.[98] The intravenous administration of IL-8 also decreases neutrophil migration to sites of inflammation.[99] Repeated intravenous administration of IL-8 causes lung injury in rats that resembles human adult respiratory distress syndrome.[100] Thus, IL-8 in PCs could potentially mediate or contribute to a variety of adverse effects, including allergic, respiratory, and even febrile reactions. However, such adverse effects may require repeated infusions or infusion in combination with significant levels of other cytokines.

Several additional observations may have relevance regarding the potential significance of cytokine levels in the supernatant fluid of blood components. First, the simultaneous presence of multiple cytokines may increase the likelihood of an adverse reaction as a result of their synergistic or additive effects. In fact, it appears that the proinflammatory cytokines are coordinately induced, ie, units with a high concentration of one cytokine are likely to have high concentrations of others. In this way, some units contain a cocktail of IL-1β, IL-6, IL-8, TNF-α, MIP-1α, GRO-α, RANTES, TGF-β, and perhaps other, as-yet-unmeasured cytokines. Several studies have demonstrated that low levels of two cytokines can act synergistically to mediate larger-than-expected responses. For example, the biologic activities of IL-1β and IL-8 may be enhanced by TNF-α.[67-69] Also, IL-1 and IL-6 can synergistically activate T lymphocytes.[70] Second, for storage-generated cytokines to be potential mediators of adverse reactions, they do not have to be detectable in all or even a majority of units at a significant level. For example, where the rate of FNHTRs is 0.5% per unit, only 1 out of every 200 units is expected to have a significant level of pyrogenic cytokines. Third, it is important to note that while several proinflammatory cytokines have been detected in the plasma portion of PCs, it cannot be determined which, if any, of these actually mediate FNHTRs or other transfusion reactions. Some are thought to be plausible candidates on the basis of correlation studies. However, the possibility exists that other, as-yet-undetected, biological response modifier(s) could also be the true causative agent(s).

Cytokine Levels Correlate With FNHTRs

If cytokines in PCs actually mediate FNHTRs, then it is expected that transfusion of PCs with high levels of proinflammatory cytokines should be associated with reactions more frequently than PCs with low levels of cytokines. In fact, such an association was observed by Muylle et al,[42] who demonstrated that the supernatant plasma of pools of PCs that caused FNHTRs more often had higher levels of IL-1β, IL-6, and TNF-α than PCs not causing reactions. Similarly, Heddle et al[40] measured higher levels of IL-1β and IL-6 in plasma from PCs that were associated with chill reactions than in plasma from PCs not associated with reactions. However, correlations do not prove that infusion of these particular cytokines causes FNHTRs because it is possible that as-yet-unmeasured biological response modifiers may be the actual causative agents.

If proinflammatory cytokines mediate FNHTRs, then elevated cytokine levels also should be detectable in the circulation of transfusion recipients experiencing reactions. Sacher and coworkers[101] assessed this by measuring intravascular IL-6 levels in the sera of patients with FNHTRs and in a group of control patients who received transfusion, but had no reaction. They found that levels of IL-6 were on average four-fold higher in the transfusion recipients having a febrile reaction. The source of the IL-6 was not determined, ie, it could have been synthesized endogenously in the recipient or it could have been produced in the blood component bags during storage, then passively infused. However, the correlation between an elevated intravascular level of a proinflammatory cytokine and an FNHTR is consistent with a role of proinflammatory cytokines in the pathogenesis of FNHTRs.

Possible Effect of the Erythrocyte Chemokine Receptor

The physiologic significance of several chemokines in transfused PCs may be affected by the erythrocyte chemokine receptor on the surface of RBCs.[102] The Duffy blood group antigens are high-affinity receptors for several chemokines, including IL-8, GRO, monocyte chemotactic protein-1 (MCP-1), and RANTES.[103,104] Individuals who are Duffy-negative, eg, have a Fy^a- or Fy^b-negative RBC phenotype, lack this chemokine receptor. The physiologic function of this receptor is not known, but may serve in vivo to bind and help clear chemokines from the circulation. The presence of this receptor possibly could bind and render inactive some of the storage-generated chemokines that are infused during platelet transfusions. Accordingly, this receptor may decrease the potential physiologic significance of IL-8, GRO-α, and RANTES from transfused PCs in Duffy-positive recipients. On the other hand, this raises the possibility that these storage-generated chemokines may have a greater potential for clinical significance in Duffy-negative recipients who lack this receptor. However, at this time, any impact of the erythrocyte chemokine receptor on the storage-generated chemokines is speculation. Moreover, no similar RBC receptor has been found for other pyrogenic proinflammatory cytokines like IL-1β, IL-6, TNF-α, or MIP-1α.

How Do Transfused Cytokines Cross the Blood-Brain Barrier?

A key question regarding the potential significance of cytokines in stored blood components is whether intravascular levels of cytokines are able to have effects on thermoregulatory centers of the brain despite the existence of the blood-brain barrier (BBB). Intravenously administrated cytokines from blood component containers must breach the BBB in some fashion in order to have their pyrogenic effects. Several mechanisms have been proposed to explain how this may be possible. As described below, these include: 1) passive transport at circumventricular organs, 2) stimulation of the cerebral vascular endothelium to generate central mediators, 3) carrier-mediated transport, and 4) activation of peripheral nerves that conduct signals centrally.

The BBB exists because of the low rate of pinocytosis in the endothelial cells and the tight junctions joining adjacent endothelial cells in the capillary beds of the brain. The BBB, however, does not exist in certain regions of the brain known as circumventricular organs. The circumventricular organs are small neuronal cell groups around the edges of the brain's ventricular system that contain fenestrated capillaries that allow neurons to come into direct contact with a variety of circulating substances.[15,17-20] Circumventricular literally means "around the ventricles" to describe their location in the brain, but circumventricular organs may also represent a means to "circumvent" the BBB. The organum vasculosum of the lamina terminalis (OVLT) is an example of a circumventricular organ. Neurons in the OVLT send efferent processes to the hypothalamus and brain stem where the centers for autonomic, endocrine, and behavioral regulation are situated. The region around the OVLT contains the highest levels of PGE_2 receptors in the brain and is the most sensitive area to fever-inducing experimental microinjections of PGE_2. In one model of fever production, circulating pyrogenic cytokines are believed to stimulate production of prostaglandins, probably of the E_2 class, by local astrocytes in circumventricular organs (Fig 2-4).[14-20] These prostaglandins in turn reach other areas of the brain, presumably through diffusion. This hypothesis is supported by experiments with systemically administered IL-1 conjugated with colloidal gold that show IL-1 localization to the OVLT, but not to other areas of the brain protected by the BBB.[105] In addition, lesions of the OVLT can block fe-

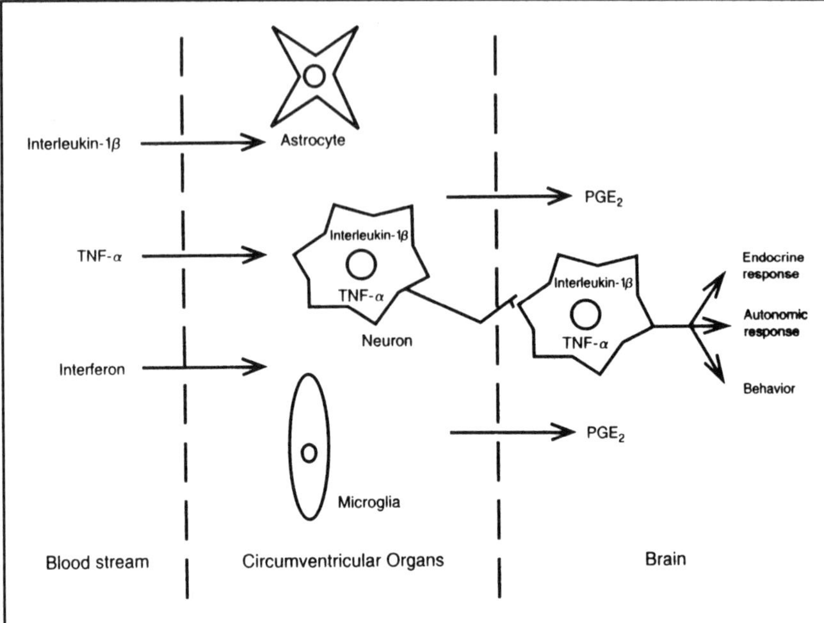

Figure 2-4. Proposed mechanism by which cytokines act across the blood-brain barrier to induce fever. Circulating cytokines enter the circumventricular organs through fenestrated capillaries, where they stimulate astrocytes, neurons, and microglia to produce prostaglandin E_2 (PGE_2). PGE_2, in turn, diffuses to thermoregulatory regions of the brain, probably in the preoptic area of the anterior hypothalamus. Alternatively, cytokines reaching the circumventricular organs may stimulate neurons to release additional cytokines or to initiate direct, neuron-neuron, signal transmission to thermoregulatory regions. TNF-α = tumor necrosis factor-alpha. (Used with permission from Saper CB and Breder CD.[14])

ver production by IL-1β, lipopolysacchride, and TNF-α.[106] Other supporting evidence shows that IL-1β can stimulate the arachidonic acid cascade, leading to the production of prostaglandins.[107] Moreover, peripheral IL-1β injections increase the level of prostaglandins in the OVLT as measured by radioimmunoassay.[108]

Circulating cytokines could also circumvent the BBB by acting directly on vascular endothelial cells, thereby either inducing the production of neuroactive substances on the brain side of the BBB or by causing a change in vascular permeability to enable larger molecules to act across the BBB.[109] The binding of IL-1β to the endothelial receptors was found to induce the production of prostaglandins, which presumably could then diffuse to other sites. Others have proposed that specific carriers transport IL-1β, IL-6, and TNF-α into the brain across the BBB.[110,111] The passage of radiolabeled IL-1β across the BBB can be inhibited by the simultaneous application of an IL-1β receptor antagonist or by the coadministration of an antibody directed against the portion of IL-1β that binds to its T-lymphocyte receptor. These data have been interpreted to indicate that passage across the BBB by IL-1β requires binding to a carrier molecule that can be inhibited by competing molecules that also bind IL-1β.

Circulating cytokines may also communicate with the central nervous system by peripheral stimulation of the vagus nerve. While the vagus itself has not been shown to express receptors for IL-1β, a chain of paraganglia closely associated with the subdiaphragmatic vagus have been shown to bind biotinylated IL-1β receptor antibody.[112,113] This chain of paraganglia may serve as chemoreceptors able to detect cytokines in the abdomen, blood, lymph, and hepatic perivascular space where liver macrophages (Kupffer cells) release cytokines in response to blood or lymph infections. Supporting evidence for this hypothesis is provided by studies that reveal the inhibitory effects of vagotomy on fever production and other centrally mediated effects of IL-1β, TNF-α, and LPS. In addition, vagotomy has been shown to reduce peripheral lipopolysaccaride-induced increases of IL-1 mRNA in the brain.[114]

Unfortunately, it is unclear at this time which, if any, of the above mechanisms accounts for the pyrogenic activity of circulating cytokines. The evidence at times seems contradictory and some investigators have argued that a blood-borne mechanism for cytokine entry into the brain does not fully explain all the experimental observations, leaving open the possibility that another mechanism may be at work.[115] Nevertheless, while the mechanisms may not be clear, it is well established that intravenous injections of recombinant human proinflammatory cytokines do have pyrogenic activity.[80,91-94] This, in turn, establishes the plausibility of pyrogenic activity for storage-generated cytokines administered intravenously in the transfusion setting.

A Model for the Pathogenesis of FNHTRs

An attempt at a unified model of an FNHTR to a variety of transfusion-related stimuli is shown in Fig 2-5. While this model is almost certainly over-simplistic, it is an attempt at a synthesis of what we currently know about FNHTRs and fever in general. It might be a framework for building future testable hypotheses concerning the pathogenesis of FNHTRs. In the

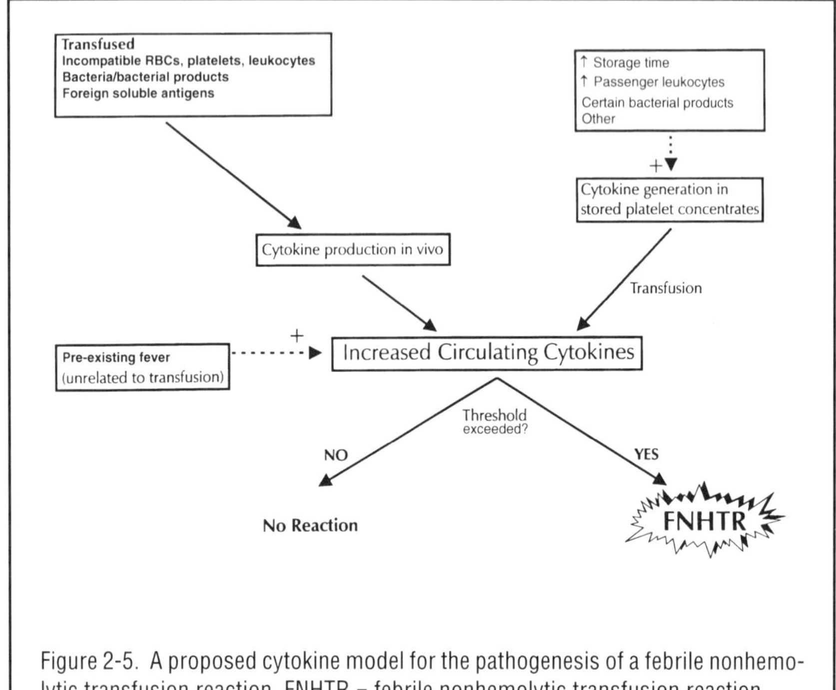

Figure 2-5. A proposed cytokine model for the pathogenesis of a febrile nonhemolytic transfusion reaction. FNHTR = febrile nonhemolytic transfusion reaction.

upper left-hand portion of the figure is shown the more "classical" pathway in which immune complexes formed in the recipient because of the infusion of immunologically incompatible RBC, platelets, leukocytes, or soluble antigens lead to the in vivo generation of cytokines in the recipient. In a similar manner, the infusion of bacteria and bacterial products can stimulate recipient monocytes to synthesize and secrete proinflammatory cytokines in vivo. If the pyrogenic cytokines reach an intravascular level that is sufficient to exceed a required threshold, then they mediate their thermoregulatory effects in the central nervous system.

The upper right-hand side of Fig 2-5 shows the pathway to FNHTRs that has more recently become evident because of the discovery of storage-generated cytokines in PCs. The amount of cytokines present in the plasma portion of PCs is affected by several variables, such as storage time of the unit, the number of passager leukocytes present, whether the unit is contaminated with certain bacteria, and other as-yet-unknown factors. After transfusion, if the level of circulating cytokines that resulted from this passive infusion exceeds the required threshold, then fever ensues.

A possible third influence on the level of circulating pyrogenic cytokines is shown on the middle left of Fig 2-5. Anecdotal reports and the "common lore" of transfusion medicine indicate that transfusion recipients who are already febrile at the start of a transfusion are at greater risk of developing an FNHTR.[25] While this is not a well-documented observation, the cytokine model of an FNHTR might provide a theoretical underpinning to support this. As a result of a preexisting fever, the transfusion recipient may already have circulating cytokines, or the pathway for fever generation may already be primed or sensitized. A precedent for such a priming effect has, in fact, been described. For example, IL-1 gene transcription can be stimulated by one signal, eg, C5a, resulting in the accumulation of intracellular, untranslated IL-1 mRNA. Small amounts of a second stimulus (eg, IL-1 itself or endotoxin) can rapidly trigger translation of this mRNA and result in more IL-1 release than would be observed from unprimed cells.[116] Perhaps in some analogous fashion, FNHTRs could more readily be induced by transfusion-related, febrile stimuli in an already primed, febrile recipient.

Cytokines and Other Adverse Effects of Transfusion

Septic Transfusion Reactions

As described earlier in the chapter, cytokines likely also mediate much of the symptomatology of septic transfusion reactions. This is supported by the demonstration by McAllister and coworkers[117] of elevated levels of proinflammatory cytokines in the plasma of patients who were transfused with RBC units contaminated with gram-negative bacilli. The greatest source of cytokines in the setting of a septic transfusion reaction is likely to be the transfusion recipient's own cells responding to the infusion of a blood component contaminated with bacteria or bacterial products. However, cytokine production in the component bag during storage stimulated by endotoxin or other bacterial products may also contribute to the reaction.[57,63] In mild cases, only a febrile reaction may ensue. In severe cases, the reaction may proceed to hypotension, shock, disseminated intravascular coagulation, multiple organ dysfunction syndrome, and death. Bacteria produce a range of extracellular products and cell wall constituents that stimulate human immune cells to produce proinflammatory cytokines. These proinflammatory and pyrogenic cytokines, such as IL-1β, IL-6, and TNF-α, are known to induce features of sepsis and septic shock.[60-62] More recently, nitric oxide produced locally within smooth muscle cells by the synergistic action of TNF-α, IL-1, and γ-interferon has emerged as a probable mediator of the refractory hypotension and vasoplegia often associated with septic shock.[118]

Allergic Transfusion Reactions

Allergic transfusion reactions are commonly attributed to the infusion of plasma proteins to which the recipient has previously made antibodies.[119] When the antibody is IgE, the resultant antigen-antibody complexes presumably directly stimulate the release of histamine from mast cells and basophils. Non-IgE antibodies presumably also mediate histamine release and allergic-type reactions via generation of the complement-derived anaphylatoxins. Elevated plasma levels of histamine have, in fact, been measured in transfusion recipients suffering from anaphylactoid reactions.[120] Several of the chemokines discovered in the plasma portions of platelet concentrates, such as IL-8, RANTES, and MIP-1α, also have the ability to recruit and activate basophils and stimulate histamine release.[7,96,121] The possibility exists, therefore, that the infusion of these cytokines present in stored PCs may also contribute to the generation of histamine and the onset of allergic-type reactions in transfusion recipients. This is a theoretical possibility that requires further investigation.

Transfusion-Related Acute Lung Injury

Transfusion-related acute lung injury (TRALI) is characterized by noncardiogenic pulmonary edema and acute respiratory distress occurring within several hours of transfusion.[122] TRALI in the majority of reported cases occurs in the setting of a passive transfer of donor HLA- or granulocyte-specific antibodies to the transfusion recipient. In an animal model, it appears that complement is a key mediator of TRALI.[123] C5a, a granulocyte chemotactic factor, appears to play a role in the migration and aggregation of granulocytes in the lung.[124] Granulocyte activation and degranulation with lysosomal enzyme release and oxygen-free radical generation may be responsible for pulmonary endothelial damage and the passage of fluid into alveolar spaces. The resultant capillary leak syndrome is the basis for the noncardiogenic pulmonary edema. Cytokines could also mediate some aspects of TRALI. IL-8, like C5a, is chemotactic for granulocytes and is emerging as a possible mediator of human acute lung injury.[125] IL-8 was reported to produce acute lung injury in laboratory animals after repeated intravenous administration.[100] Theoretically and based on animal models, the repeated infusion of IL-8 in blood components could contribute to TRALI-like symptoms. In addition, TNF could theoretically contribute to the development of a TRALI-like syndrome because acute respiratory distress has been reported as a side effect of the intravenous administration of recombinant TNF.[93]

Other Adverse Effects

Other adverse effects to the infusion of cytokines in stored blood components are possible. For example, it is theoretically possible that proinflammatory cytokines in PCs may affect the replication of human immunodeficiency virus-1 (HIV-1). The chemokines MIP-1α and RANTES are known to inhibit HIV-1 replication, whereas TNF-α, IL-1β, and IL-6 upregulate HIV-1 replication.[126-128] MIP-1α and RANTES inhibit HIV-1 infection by interfering with the virus-cell fusion reaction that requires the β-chemokine CCR-5 receptor.[128] Cytokines might affect HIV-1 replication either in the transfusion recipient or in the blood component container. However, it is difficult to predict the net effect, if any, that storage-related cytokines might have because of the counteracting effects that the various cytokines generated in PCs can have on HIV-1 replication. Since cytokines have such a wide range of biologic activities, an effect on virus replication is only one of a variety of other possible effects of storage-generated cytokines. Elucidation of these other possible effects awaits the outcome of future research.

Summary

Based on an understanding of the role that proinflammatory cytokines play in the pathogenesis of fever and inflammatory syndromes, it is expected that cytokines also play a significant role in the etiology of FNHTRs and possibly other types of transfusion reactions. One source of proinflammatory cytokines in the transfusion setting is likely to be the transfusion recipient's own cells. However, physiologically significant levels of cytokines also appear to be generated during the blood bank storage of some cellular blood components, particularly PCs. These storage-generated cytokines may account for a variety of previously unexplained observations regarding the relationship between FNHTRs and PCs, such as: 1) reaction to a first transfusion in patients not previously alloimmunized to leukocytes, 2) failure of bedside leukocyte reduction to prevent FNHTRs, 3) increased frequency of FNHTRs to PCs stored for longer periods, and 4) the ability of the supernatant plasma portion of PCs to induce chill reactions. To support a role of storage-generated cytokines in the pathogenesis of FNHTRs, evidence exists that levels of proinflammatory cytokines are higher in PCs that cause FNHTRs. Also, levels of at least one cytokine, IL-6, are elevated in transfusion recipients suffering from FNHTRs. The source of most of the cytokines with pyrogenic activity appears to be the passenger leukocytes in cellular blood components. The best evidence at this time indicates that the accumulation of leukocyte-derived cytokines during the storage of PCs is due to new synthesis and secretion, rather than cell disruption and leakage. The accumulation of leukoctye-derived cytokines during blood component storage is inhibited by prestorage or early-storage filter leukocyte reduction and by lower storage temperatures. Further study is required to determine whether these or any other methods for preventing cytokine generation during blood component storage will prove effective in decreasing FNHTRs.

References

1. Paul WE, Seder RA. Lymphocyte responses and cytokines. Cell 1994;76:241-51.
2. Bellanti JA, Kadlec JV, Escobar GA. Cytokines and the immune response. Pediatr Clin North Am 1994;41:597-621.
3. Rees RC. Cytokines as biological response modifiers. J Clin Pathol 1992;45:93-8.
4. Janeway CA, Travers P. Immunobiology. New York, NY: Garland Publishing, 1994:12-21.
5. Kelvin DJ, Michiel DF, Johnston JA, et al. Chemokines and serpentines: The molecular biology of chemokine receptors. J Leukoc Biol 1993;54:604-12.
6. Ahuja SK, Gao J-L, Murphy PM. Chemokine receptors and molecular mimicry. Immunol Today 1994;15:281-7.
7. Baggiolini M, Dahinden CA. CC chemokines in allergic inflammation. Immunol Today 1994;15:127-33.
8. Heinrich PC, Castell JV, Andus T. Interleukin-6 and the acute phase response. Biochem J 1990;265:621-36.
9. Bone RC. Toward an epidemiology and natural history of SIRS (systemic inflammatory response syndrome). JAMA 1992;268:3452-5.
10. Beal AL, Cerra FB. Multiple organ failure syndrome in the 1990s: Systemic inflammatory response and organ dysfunction. JAMA 1994;271:226-33.
11. Menkin V. Chemical basis of fever with inflammation. Arch Pathol 1945;39:28-36.
12. Bennett ILJ, Beeson PB. Studies on the pathogenesis of fever. II. Characterization of fever-producing substances from polymorphonuclear leukocytes and from the fluid of sterile exudates. J Exp Med 1953;98:493-508.
13. Dinarello CA. Endogenous pyrogens. Methods Enzymol 1988; 163:495-510.

14. Saper CB, Breder CD. The neurologic basis of fever. N Engl J Med 1994;330:1880-6.
15. Kapás L, Shibata M, Krueger JM. Role of cytokines in sleep, fever, and anorexia. In: Aggarwal BB, Puri RK, eds. Human cytokines: Their role in disease and therapy. Cambridge, MA: Blackwell Scientific, 1995:305-14.
16. Dinarello CA, Cannon JG, Wolff SM. New concepts on the pathogenesis of fever. Rev Infect Dis 1988,10:168-89.
17. Blatteis CM. Neuromodulative actions of cytokines. Yale J Biol Med 1990;63:133-46.
18. Shibata M. Hypothalamic neuronal responses to cytokines. Yale J Biol Med 1990;63:147-56.
19. Stitt JT. Passage of immunomodulators across the blood-brain barrier. Yale J Biol Med 1990;63:121-31.
20. Zeisberger E, Roth J. Neurobiological concepts of fever generation and suppression. Neuropsychobiology 1993;28:106-9.
21. Davatelis G, Wolpe SD, Sherry B, et al. Macrophage inflammatory protein-1: A prostaglandin-independent endogenous pyrogen. Science 1989;243:1066-8.
22. Heddle NM, Kelton JG. Febrile nonhemolytic transfusion reactions. In: Popovsky MA, ed. Transfusion reactions. Bethesda, MD: AABB Press, 1996:45-80.
23. Stack G, Judge JV, Snyder EL. Febrile and nonimmune transfusion reactions. In: Rossi EC, Simon TL, Moss GS, Gould SA, eds. Principles of transfusion medicine, 2nd ed. Baltimore, MD: Williams and Wilkins, 1995:773-84.
24. Perkins HA, Payne R, Ferguson J, Wood M. Nonhemolytic febrile transfusion reactions. Quantitative effects of blood components with emphasis on isoantigenic incompatibility of leukoctyes. Vox Sang 1966;11:578-600.
25. Walker RH. Special report: Transfusion risks. Am J Clin Pathol 1987;88:374-8.
26. Menitove JE, McElligott MC, Aster RH. Febrile transfusion reaction: What blood component should be given next? Vox Sang 1982;42: 318-21.
27. Chambers LA, Kruskall MS, Pacini DG, Donovan LM. Febrile reactions after platelet transfusion: The effect of single versus multiple donors. Transfusion 1990;30:212-21.

28. Lane TA, Anderson KC, Goodnough LT, et al. Leukocyte reduction in blood component therapy. Ann Intern Med 1992;117:151-62.
29. Decary F, Ferner P, Giavedoni L, et al. An investigation of nonhemolytic transfusion reactions. Vox Sang 1984;46:277-85.
30. de Rie MA, van der Plas-van Dalen CM, Engelfriet CP, von dem Borne AE. The serology of febrile transfusion reactions. Vox Sang 1985;49:126-34.
31. Heinrich D, Mueller-Eckhardt C, Stier W. The specificity of leukocyte and platelet alloantibodies in sera of patients with nonhemolytic tranfusion reactions. Vox Sang 1973;25:442-56.
32. Brubaker DB. Clinical significance of white cell antibodies in febrile nonhemolytic transfusion reactions. Transfusion 1990;30:733-7.
33. Killman SA. Febrile transfusion reactions in patients with leukocyte agglutinins. Dan Med Bull 1958;5:178-83.
34. Brittingham TE, Chaplin H Jr. Febrile transfusion reactions caused by sensitivity to donor leukocytes and platelets. JAMA 1957;165:819-25.
35. Payne R. The association of febrile transfusion reactions with leukoagglutinins. Vox Sang 1957;2:233-41.
36. Mangano MM, Chambers LA, Kruskall MS. Limited efficacy of leukopoor platelets for prevention of febrile transfusion reactions. Am J Clin Pathol 1991;95:733-8.
37. Goodnough LT, Riddell J IV, Lazarus H, et al. Prevalence of platelet transfusion reactions before and after implementation of leukocyte-depleted platelet concentrates by filtration. Vox Sang 1993;65:103-7.
38. Muylle L, Wouters E, De Bock R, et al. Reactions to platelet transfusion: The effect of the storage time of the concentrates. Transfus Med 1992;2:289-93.
39. Heddle NM, Klama LN, Griffith L, et al. A prospective study to identify the risk factors associated with acute reactions to platelet and red cell transfusions. Transfusion 1993;33:794-7.
40. Heddle NM, Klama L, Singer J. The role of plasma from platelet concentrates in transfusion reactions. N Engl J Med 1994;331:625-8.
41. Stack G, Snyder EL. Interleukin-8 generation in platelet concentrates during storage (abstract). Blood 1991;78(Suppl):388a.
42. Muylle L, Joos M, Wouters E, et al. Increased tumor necrosis factor α (TNFα), interleukin 1, and interleukin 6 (IL-6) levels in the plasma of stored platelet concentrates: Relationship between TNF-α and IL-6 levels and febrile transfusion reactions. Transfusion 1993;33:195-9.

43. Stack G, Snyder EL. Cytokine generation in stored platelet concentrates. Transfusion 1994;34:20-5.
44. Aye MT, Palmer DS, Giulivi A, Hashemi S. Effect of filtration on platelet concentrates on the accumulation of cytokines and platelet release factors during storage. Transfusion 1995;35:117-24.
45. Cole S, Stack G. Macrophage inflammatory protein-1α generation in stored platelets (abstract). Blood 1993; 82 (Suppl):398a.
46. Cole S, Stack G. Accumulation of the chemokine GRO-α in stored, leukoreduced and bacterially contaminated platelet concentrates (abstract). Am J Clin Pathol 1995;104:223.
47. Stack G, Cole S. Accumulation of the cytokines TGF-β_1 and RANTES in stored platelet concentrates (abstract). Transfusion 1995;35 (Suppl):45S.
48. Bubel S, Wilhelm D, Entelmann M, et al. Chemokines in stored platelet concentrates. Transfusion 1996;36:445-9.
49. Klinger MHF, Wilhelm D, Bubel S, et al. Immunocytochemical localization of the chemokines RANTES and MIP-1α within human platelets and their release during storage. Int Arch Allergy Immunol 1995;107:541-6.
50. Stack G. Cytokine accumulation in stored platelet concentrates: Detection, prevention, and potential significance. Biol Clin Hematol 1995;17:58-64.
51. Stack G, Snyder EL. Leukodepletion to prevent transfusion reactions: Effects on cytokines and other biologic response modifiers. In: Sweeney J, Heaton A, eds. Clinical benefits of leukodepleted blood products. Austin, TX: RG Landes, 1994:61-80.
52. Kluter H, Muller-Steinhardt M, Danzer S, et al. Cytokines in platelet concentrates prepared from pooled buffy coats. Vox Sang 1995;69: 38-43.
53. Flegel WA, Wiesneth M, Stampe D, Koerner K. Low cytokine contamination in buffy coat-derived platelet concentrates without filtration. Transfusion 1995;35:917-20.
54. Sweeney JD, Holme S, Moroff G. Storage of apheresis platelets after gamma radiation. Transfusion 1994;34:779-83.
55. Shimizu T, Vehigiri C, Mizuno S, et al. Adsorption of anaphylatoxins and platelet-specific proteins by filtration of platelet concentrates with a polyester leukocyte-reduction filter. Vox Sang 1994;66:161-5.
56. Muylle L, Peetermans ME. Effect of prestorage leukocyte removal on the cytokine levels in stored platelet concentrates. Vox Sang 1994;66:14-7.

57. Stack G, Baril L, Napychank P, Snyder EL. Cytokine generation in stored, white cell-reduced, and bacterially-contaminated units of red blood cells. Transfusion 1995;35:199-203.
58. Heddle N, Tan M, Klama L, Shroeder J. Factors affecting cytokine production in platelet concentrates (abstract). Transfusion 1994;34 (Suppl):67S.
59. Sriskandan S, Cohen J. The pathogenesis of septic shock. J Infect Dis 1995;30:201-6.
60. Levi M, ten Cate H, van der Poll T, et al. Pathogenesis of disseminated intravascular coagulation in sepsis. JAMA 1993;270:975-9.
61. Dofferhoff ASM, Bom VJJ, de Vries-Hospers HG, et al. Patterns of cytokines, plasma endotoxin, plasminogen activator inhibitor, and acute-phase proteins during the treatment of severe sepsis in humans. Crit Care Med 1992;20:185-92.
62. Martich GD, Danner RL, Ceska M, Suffredini AF. Detection of interleukin-8 and tumor necrosis factor in normal humans after intravenous endotoxin: The effect of antiinflammatory agents. J Exp Med 1991;173:1021-4.
63. Stack G, Cole S, Campbell S, et al. Interleukin-8 generation in bacterially contaminated platelet concentrates (abstract). Transfusion 1993;33(Suppl):50S.
64. Chao T-C, Van Alten PJ, Greager JA, Walter RJ. Steroid sex hormones regulate the release of tumor necrosis factor by macrophages. Cell Immunol 1995;160:43-9.
65. Takahashi TA, Fujihara M, Ogiso C, et al. Cytokine level determination in stored apheresis platelet concentrates (abstract). Transfusion 1995;35(Suppl):44S.
66. Smith KJ, Sierra ER, Nelson EJ. Histamine, IL-1β, and IL-8 increase in packed RBCs stored for 42 days but not in RBCs leukodepleted pre-storage (abstract). Transfusion 1993;33(Suppl):53S.
67. Yuo A, Kitagawa S, Kasahara T, et al. Stimulation and priming of human neutrophils by interleukin-8: Cooperation with tumor necrosis factor and colony stimulating factors. Blood 1991;78:2708-14.
68. Elias JA, Gustilo K, Baeder W, Freundlich B. Synergistic stimulation of fibroblast prostaglandin by recombinant interleukin 1 and tumor necrosis factor. J Immunol 1987;138:3812-6.
69. Okusawa S, Gelfond JA, Ikejima T, et al. Interleukin 1 induces a shock-like state in rabbits. Synergism with tumor necrosis factor and the effect of cyclo oxygenase inhibition. J Clin Invest 1988;8:1162-72.

70. Houssiau FA, Coulie PG, Olive D, et al. Synergistic activation of human T-cells by interleukin 1 and interleukin 6. Eur J Immunol 1988;18:653-8.
71. Fuhlbrigge RC, Chaplin DD, Kiely J-M, Unanue ER. Regulation of interleukin-1 gene expression by adherence and lipopolysaccharide. J Immunol 1987;138:3799-802.
72. Kasahara K, Strieter RM, Chensure SW, et al. Mononuclear cell adherence induces neutrophil chemotactic factor/interleukin-8 gene expression. J Leukoc Biol 1991;50:287-95.
73. Eierman DF, Johnson CE, Haskill JS. Human monocyte inflammatory mediator gene expression is selectively regulated by adherence substrates. J Immunol 1989;142:1970-6.
74. Elkattan I, Anderson J, Yun JK, et al. Mononuclear cell (MC) adhesion to platelet storage bag plastic polymers correlates with cytokine levels (abstract). Transfusion 1995;35(Suppl):44S.
75. Rinder HM, Snyder EL. Activation of platelet concentrate during preparation and storage. Blood Cells 1992;18:445-56.
76. Weyrich AS, Elstad MR, McEver RP, et al. Activated platelets signal chemokine synthesis by human monocytes. J Clin Invest 1996;97:1525-34.
77. Miletic VD, Popovic O. Complement activation in stored platelet concentrates. Transfusion 1993;33:150-4.
78. Schleuning M, Böck M, Mempel W. Complement activation during storage of single-donor platelet concentrates. Vox Sang 1994;67:144-8.
79. Okusawa S, Dinarello CA, Endres S, et al. C5a induction of human interleukin-1: Synergistic effect with endotoxin or interferon-α. J Immunol 1987;139:2635-40.
80. Dinarello CA. Interleukin-1 and interleukin-1 antagonism. Blood 1991;77:1627-52.
81. Fracasso A, Calo L, Landini S, et al. Peritoneal sclerosis: Role of plasticizers in stimulating interleukin-1 production. Perit Dial Int 1993;13:S517-9.
82. Metinko AP, Kunkel SL, Sandiford TJ, Strieter RM. Anoxia-hyperoxia induces monocyte driven IL-8. J Clin Invest 1992;90: 791-8.
83. Karakurum M, Shreeniwas R, Chen J et al. Hypoxic induction of interleukin-8 gene expression in human endothelial cells. J Clin Invest 1994;93:1564-70.

84. Jessop JJ, Hoffman T. Production and release of IL-1β by human peripheral blood monocytes in response to diverse stimuli: Possible role of "microdamage" to account for unregulated release. Lymphokine Cytokine Res 1993;12:51-8.
85. Hogquist K, Nett MA, Unanue ER, Chaplin DD. Interleukin 1 is processed and released during apoptosis. Proc Natl Acad Sci USA 1991;88:8485-89.
86. Dinarello CA, Cannon JG, Wolff SM, et al. Tumor necrosis factor (cachectin) is an endogenous pyrogen and induces production of interleukin 1. J Exp Med 1986;163:1433-50.
87. Van Zee KJ, DeForge LE, Fischer E, et al. IL-8 in septic shock, endotoxemia and after IL-1 administration. J Immunol 1991;146:3478-82.
88. Streiter RM, Kunkel SL, Showell HJ, et al. Endothelial cell gene expression of a neutrophil chemotactic factor by TNF-α, LPS, and IL-1β. Science 1989;243:1467-9.
89. Schindler R, Mancilla J, Endres S, et al. Correlations and interactions in the production of interleukin 6 (IL-6), IL-1, and tumor necrosis factor (TNF) in human blood mononuclear cells: IL-6 suppresses IL-1 and TNF. Blood 1990;75:40-7.
90. Chantry D, Turner M, Abney E, Feldmann M. Modulation of cytokine production by transforming growth factor-beta. J Immunol 1989;142:4295-300.
91. Tewari A, Buhles WC Jr, Starnes HF Jr. Preliminary report: Effects of interleukin-1 on platelet counts. Lancet 1990;336:712-4.
92. Crown J, Jakubowski A, Kemeny N, et al. A phase I trial of recombinant human interleukin-1β alone and in combination with myelosuppressive doses of 5-fluorouracil in patients with gastrointestinal cancer. Blood 1991;78:1420-7.
93. Schiller JH, Storer BE, Witt PL, et al. Biological and clinical effects of intravenous tumor necrosis factor-alpha administered three times weekly. Cancer Res 1991;51:1651-8.
94. Agosti JM, Coombs RW, Collier AC, et al. A randomized, double-blind, phase I/II trial of tumor necrosis factor and interferon-gamma for treatment of AIDS-related complex (Protocol 025 from the AIDS Clinical Trials Group). AIDS Res Hum Retroviruses 1992;8:581-7.
95. Baggiolini M, Clark Lewis I. Interleukin-8, a chemotactic and inflammatory cytokine. FEBS Lett 1992;307:97-101.

96. Dahinden CA, Kurimoto Y, De Wech AL, et al. The neutrophil activating peptide NAF/NAP-1 induces histamine and leukotriene release by interleukin 3-primed basophils. J Exp Med 1989;170:1787-92.
97. Hack CE, Hart M, Van Schijndel RJ, et al. Interleukin-8 in sepsis: Relation to shock and inflammatory mediators. Infect Immun 1992;60: 2835-42.
98. Van Zee KJ, Fischer E, Hawes AS, et al. Effects of intravenous IL-8 administration in non-human primates. J Immunol 1992;148:1746-52.
99. Hechtman DH, Cybulsky M, Fuchs HJ, et al. Intravascular IL-8. Inhibitor of polymorphonuclear leukocyte accumulation at sites of acute inflammation. J Immunol 1991;147:883-92.
100. Rot A. Some aspects of NAP-1 pathophysiology: Lung damage caused by a blood-borne cytokine. Adv Exp Med Biol 1991;305: 127-35.
101. Sacher RA, Boyle L, Freter CE. High circulating interleukin 6 levels associated with acute transfusion reaction: Cause or effect? (letter). Transfusion 1993;33:962.
102. Horuk R, Chitnis CE, Darbonne WC, et al. A receptor for the malarial parasite *Plasmodium vivax*: The erythrocyte chemokine receptor. Science 1993;261:1182-4.
103. Neote K, Darbonne W, Ogez J, et al. Identification of a promiscuous inflammatory peptide receptor on the surface of red blood cells. J Biol Chem 1993;268:12247-9.
104. Chaudhuri A, Zbrzezna V, Polyskova J, et al. Expression of the Duffy antigen in K562 cells. J Biol Chem 1994;269:7835-8.
105. Hashimoto M, Ishikawa Y, Yokota S, et al. Action site of circulating interleukin-1 on the rabbit brain. Brain Res Bull 1991;540:217-23.
106. Blatteis CM, Bealer SL, Hunter WS, et al. Suppression of fever after lesions of the anteroventral third ventricle in guinea pigs. Brain Res Bull 1983;11:519-26.
107. Katsuura G, Gottschall PE, Dahl RR, Arimura A. Interleukin-1 beta increases prostaglandin E2 in rat astrocyte cultures: Modulatory effect of neuropeptides. Endocrinology 1989;124:3125-7.
108. Komaki G, Arimura A, Koves K. Effect of intravenous injection of IL-1 beta on PGE_2 levels in several brain areas as determined by microdialysis. Am J Physiol 1992;262:E246-51.
109. Maier JA, Voulalas P, Roeder D, Maciag T. Extension of the life-span of human endothelial cells by an interleukin-1 alpha antisense oligomer. Science 1990;249:1570-4.

110. Banks WA, Kastin AJ. Saturable transport of peptides across the blood-brain barrier. Life Sci 1987;41:1319-38.
111. Banks WA, Kastin AJ. Blood to brain transport of interleukin links the immune and central nervous systems. Life Sci 1991;48:PL117-21.
112. Morgan M, Pack RJ, Howe A. Structure of cells and nerve endings in abdominal vagal paraganglia of the rat. Cell Tissue Res 1976;169: 467-84.
113. Berthoud HR, Powley TL. Characterization of vagal innervation to the rat celiac, suprarenal and mesenteric ganglia. J Auton Nerv Syst 1993;42:153-69.
114. Laye S, Bluthe RM, Kent S, et al. Subdiaphragmatic vagotomy blocks induction of IL-1 beta mRNA in mice brain in response to peripheral LPS. Am J Physiol 1995;268:R1327-31.
115. Watkins LR, Maier SF, Goehler LE. Cytokine-to-brain communication: A review and analysis of alternative mechanisms. Life Sci 1995;57:1011-26.
116. Schindler R, Gelfand JA, Dinarello CA. Recombinant C5a stimulates transcription rather than translation of interleukin-1 (IL-1) and tumor necrosis factor: Translational signal provided by lipopolysaccharide or IL-1 itself. Blood 1990;76:1631-8.
117. McAllister SK, Bland LA, Arduino MJ, et al. Patient cytokine response in transfusion-associated sepsis. Infect Immunol 1994;62:2126-8.
118. Cobb JP, Danner RL. Nitric oxide and septic shock. JAMA 1996;275: 1192-6.
119. Vamvakas EC, Pineda AA. Allergic and anaphylactic reactions. In: Popovsky MA, ed. Transfusion reactions. Bethesda, MD: AABB Press, 1996:81-123.
120. Frewin DB, Jonsson JR, Frewin CR, et al. Influence of blood storage time and plasma histamine levels on the pattern of transfusion reactions. Vox Sang 1989;56:243-6.
121. Kuna P, Reddigari SR, Schall TJ, et al. RANTES, a monocyte and T lymphocyte chemotactic cytokine releases histamine from human basophils. J Immunol 1992;149:636-42.
122. Popovsky MA, Moore SB. Diagnostic and pathogenetic considerations in transfusion-related acute lung injury. Transfusion 1985;25: 573-7.
123. Seeger W, Schneider U, Kreusler B, et al. Reproduction of transfusion-related acute lung injury in an ex vivo lung model. Blood 1990;76: 1438-44.

124. Jacob HS, Craddock PR, Hammerschmidt DE, Moldow CF. Complement-induced granulocyte aggregation: An unsuspected mechanism of disease. N Engl J Med 1980;302:789-94.
125. Kunkel SL, Standiford T, Kasahara K, Strieter RM. Interleukin-8 (IL-8): The major neutrophil chemotactic factor in the lung. Exp Lung Res 1991;17:17-23.
126. Cocchi F, DeVico AL, Garzino-Demo A, et al. Identification of RANTES, MIP-1α, and MIP-1β as the major HIV-suppressive factors produced by CD8+ T cells. Science 1995;270:1811-5.
127. Poli G, Fauci AS. Role of cytokines in the pathogenesis of human immunodeficiency virus infection. In: Aggarwal BB, Puri RD, eds. Human cytokines: Their role in disease and therapy. Cambridge, MA: Blackwell, 1995:421-49.
128. Dragic T, Litwin V, Allaway GP, et al. HIV-1 entry into CD4+ cells is mediated by the chemokine receptor CC-CKR-5. Nature 1996;381:667-73.

In: Davenport RD, Snyder EL, eds.
Cytokines in Transfusion Medicine: A Primer
Bethesda, MD: AABB Press, 1997

3

Biological Response Modifiers in Blood Component Processing

TERRENCE L. GEIGER, MD, PhD, AND
EDWARD L. SNYDER, MD

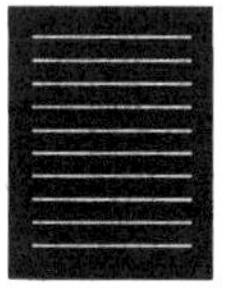

BIOLOGICAL RESPONSE MODIFIERS (BRMS) ARE A DIVERSE group of molecules that include chemokines, interleukins, complement fragments, arachidonic acid metabolites, kininogens, enzymes, and an array of other biologically active organic and inorganic compounds (Table 3-1). BRMs share the ability to alter cellular physiology through their interactions with cellular and humoral receptors.

As the mechanisms by which BRMs function have become apparent, their role in human disease pathogenesis has become increasingly clear.

Terrence L. Geiger, MD, PhD, Fellow, Yale University School of Medicine; and Edward L. Snyder, MD, Professor of Laboratory Medicine, Yale University School of Medicine, School, and Director, Blood Bank and Apheresis, Yale-New Haven Hospital, New Haven, Connecticut

Table 3-1. Biological Response Modifiers Suspected of Mediating Adverse Reactions to Transfused Blood Components

Biological Response Modifier	Source	Activities
IL-I	Macrophage Epithelial cells	Fever Macrophage/T-cell activation
IL-6	T cells Macrophage	Acute phase reactant T- and B-cell growth/ differentiation
IL-8	Macrophage Other cell types	Neutrophil/T-cell chemotaxin
TNF-α	Macrophage NK cells	Fever Local inflammation Endothelial activation
RANTES	T cells Platelets	Monocyte/T cell/eosinophil Chemoattractant
C3a	Plasma precursor	Increased vascular permeability Mast cell/basophil degranulation
C5a	Plasma precursor	Leukocyte chemotaxin Mast cell/basophil degranulation
Histamine	Basophils/mast cells Platelets	Vasodilatation Increased capillary permeability
Bradykinin	Plasma precursor	Vasodilatation

IL = interleukin; TNF-α = tumor necrosis factor alpha; NK = natural killer.

BRMs have been implicated as critical mediators of sepsis, acute respiratory distress syndrome, and multiorgan failure.[1,2] They also have been documented to promote adverse effects in cancer syndromes, autoimmune states, and a variety of other conditions.[3-6]

A growing body of data shows that BRMs formed in blood or blood components ex vivo and infused into a host can be harmful.[7] BRMs generated ex vivo may induce anaphylactoid reactions, neutrophil and platelet activation, capillary leak syndrome, myocardial depression, and febrile transfusion reactions.[8-14] Some evidence implicates anaphylatoxins, such as C3a and C5a, as well as cytokines, such as interleukin-1 beta (IL-1β), interleukin-6 (IL-6), interleukin-8 (IL-8), and tumor necrosis factor-alpha (TNF-α). Other data suggest a role for the kininogens, as they degrade releasing bradykinin.[15,16] The fact that only a limited number of BRMs have been implicated in these responses likely reflects the limited data thus far collected. As our understanding of the ex-vivo formation of BRMs evolves, the importance of other BRMs, such as the arachidonic acid metabolites, will likely become clearer.

Ex-vivo BRM formation is particularly important in transfusion medicine. Bioincompatible polymer surfaces, such as those found in plastic blood storage bags, promote BRM formation by activating leukocytes, platelets, complement, and other plasma enzyme cascades.[17-20] Furthermore, physiologic means for disposing of BRMs are not available in closed blood storage systems. Consequently, high levels of BRMs can accumulate in a blood component and, if infused into a patient, can produce adverse effects.[7] Thus, prevention of BRM formation and removal of BRMs in blood components have become a major focus in transfusion biology.

Leukocyte reduction (LR) filters are known to play a direct role in the formation and elimination of some BRMs in blood components.[16,21-23] These filters have assumed an increasingly prominent role in transfusion medicine because of their ability to remove white blood cells.[24] Indeed, leukocyte reduction has been shown to decrease the incidence of febrile transfusion reactions, alloimmunization, and the transmission of cytomegalovirus (CMV) and some other infectious diseases.[25] Because the benefits of LR filters primarily relate to their efficiency in removing leukocytes, their role in BRM formation and elimination has generally not been fully considered in filter design and fabrication. This chapter reviews the available data on the formation and removal of BRMs in blood components with an emphasis on the role of LR filters.

Complement Activation in Blood Components

The complement system is composed of a series of plasma proteins that form an enzymatic cascade (Fig 3-1).[26-28] Complement provides a first line of defense against pathogens. Two activation pathways exist: the classical pathway and the alternative pathway. The classical pathway is especially

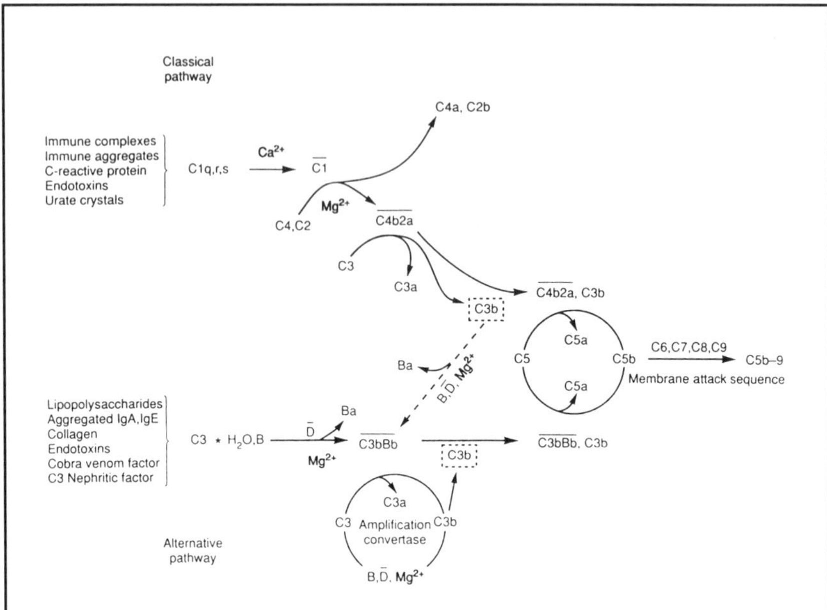

Figure 3-1. Reaction scheme of the complement activation pathways. Components displaying enzymatic activity are denoted by a solid bar above the symbol. C3H^{2}0 is generated from C3 by spontaneous hydrolysis of an internal thiol ester bond in the C3a chain. The dashed arrow denotes the crossover between classic and alternative pathways, through which C3b generated by the classic pathway C3-convertase ($\overline{C4b2a}$) serves as the membrane cofactor for assembly of the alternative pathway C3-convertase ($\overline{C3bBb}$). Also note the potential for self-propagation of the $\overline{C3bBb}$ enzyme complex through the cycle of the amplication convertase. (Used with permission from Sims.[28])

sensitive to immunoglobulin multimers and antigen-antibody complexes. The alternative pathway, while sensitive to immune complexes, recognizes bacterial lipopolysaccharide, yeast cell walls, some virus membranes, biopolymers, and other biomaterial surfaces. Activation of complement can induce a variety of effector responses. If activation of the complement cascade is complete, a membrane attack complex containing C5b-9 is formed. This membrane attack complex creates a water channel that is an actual membrane pore, promoting osmotic rupture of a targeted cell.

Complement activation, however, is not always complete. Soluble and cell surface proteins downmodulate the complement system, preventing its uncontrolled activation (Fig 3-1). These regulatory proteins include C1-

INH, which blocks the enzymatic activity of activated C1 fragments; Factor H, which inhibits the association of C3b with Factor B and promotes C3b degradation; C4b-binding protein, which blocks the association of C4b with C2; CD55 (decay accelerating factor), which promotes the dissociation of membrane-associated $\overline{\text{C4b2a}}$ and $\overline{\text{C3bBb}}$; vitronectin (S-protein), which prevents cell-to-cell transfer of membrane attack complexes by binding newly formed C5b67; and CD59 (homologous restriction factor), which prevents formation of the membrane attack complex by inhibiting poly C9 binding to membrane-bound C5b678.

Even in the absence of membrane attack complex formation, activated early complement components can enhance the opsonization of foreign particles, prevent immune complex deposition, and promote inflammation. Among such early products of complement activation are the anaphylatoxins C3a, C4a, and C5a (26, 27). C3a and C4a seem to bind the same cellular receptor. Activation induces the degranulation of mast cells and basophils, release of vasoactive molecules, such as histamine, and an increase in vascular permeability. C5a, which is approximately 10-fold more potent than C3a, binds to a distinct cell surface receptor. In addition to stimulating mast cell and basophil degranulation, C5a stimulates neutrophil and mononuclear cell chemotaxis, increases neutrophil adhesiveness and opsonization, and stimulates neutrophil respiratory activity. The activities of C3a and C5a are limited by carboxypeptidases N and R, which remove their N-terminal arginine. Whereas C5a-des-arg has limited biologic activity, C3a-des-arg has essentially none.

Activated complement has long been suspected in the adverse effects associated with extracorporeal circulation systems, such as cardiopulmonary bypass and hemodialysis. These effects include platelet and neutrophil activation, neutropenia, myocardial compromise, adult respiratory distress syndrome, and anaphylactoid reactions.[9,29-32] Presumably, complement activation is the result of the passage of blood over bioincompatible surfaces. Alternative pathway activation results when surface-associated C3 is activated and associates with protein B to form the C3 convertase $\overline{\text{C3bBb}}$ or the C3/C5 convertase complex $\overline{\text{C3bBb}}$•C3b.[18] This activates the remainder of the complement cascade, resulting in the formation of the C5b-9 membrane attack complex (Fig 3-1).

In contrast to extracorporeal circuits, which usually rely on heparin as an anticoagulant, citrate serves as the anticoagulant in stored blood components.[33] Because citrate binds the divalent cations calcium and magnesium, necessary cofactors in the complement enzymatic cascade, it would be expected that complement would not be activated in citrated blood components. However, the generation of anaphylatoxins in both stored platelet concentrates and whole blood has been well documented.[33,34] Hence, although magnesium and calcium promote anaphylatoxin formation, they may not be essential or may be present at functional levels even in the presence of chelating agents. This is further supported by one report that described studies of complement activation by cellulose acetate filters.[18] Even in the presence of ethylenediaminetetraacetic acid (EDTA), which binds divalent cations such as magnesium and calcium more strongly than citrate, 30% of the C3 activation present in the absence of any chelator is observed.

Complement activation in blood components is presumed to result from the interaction of plasma with plastic surfaces and not from leukocyte-mediated activation. Indeed, Gyongossy-Issa et al showed greater levels of C4d, C5a, and SC5b-9 in stored platelet-poor plasma than in platelet concentrates that were rich in leukocytes.[20] Complement activation was observed after storage in both polyvinyl chloride (PVC)/tri (2-ethyl-hexyl) trimelliate (TOTM) and polyolefin bags.

The degree of complement activation in conventionally stored blood components may be high. In one study of complement activation in platelet concentrates, complement-mediated inhibition of immune precipitation was completely lost in many units after 5 days of storage. A lesser degree of activation was observed by using the generation of C3 activation products or complement-mediated hemolysis as outcome measures.[35]

Complement activation in stored blood components can have several effects. Activated complement components can activate platelets, an event that some believe potentiates the development of platelet storage lesion.[20,29,36,37] This may occur by enhancing platelet microparticle formation, increasing platelet prothrombinase activity, and increasing platelet sensitivity to agonists.[29,38,39] Likewise, activated complement components, such as C3b, are potent opsonins. By promoting phagocytosis of transfused platelets, the opsonins may decrease platelet lifespan. Activated complement can also activate leukocytes, which promote the release of IL-1 and possibly other cytokines.[30] Transfusion of blood components with high levels of these cytokines has been associated with febrile transfusion reactions.[7,40]

It is not known whether transfused anaphylatoxins and activated complement can directly mediate pathologic reactions. In most circumstances, these substances will be rapidly diluted in the recipient's circulation or inactivated by complement inhibitors. However, sometimes this may not be the case. In the massively transfused patient, large quantities of anaphylatoxins and activated complement may be transfused while complement inhibitors are diluted. In patients with autoimmune hemolytic anemias, transfusion of activated complement may promote hemolysis. Case reports document enhanced hemolysis after transfusion in patients with cold autoimmune hemolytic anemia.[41] This is presumed to result from transfusion of complement proteins in complement-depleted individuals. Although definitive evidence is lacking, similar susceptibility to transfused complement would be expected in patients with deficiencies in complement inhibitor function, such as paroxysmal nocturnal hemoglobinuria (PNH). There are reported cases of hemolysis following transfusion in PNH patients; however, one study suggests that PNH patients do not benefit from receiving red blood cells washed with saline before transfusion (an action expected to remove complement proteins).[42]

Complement activation may be particularly high in wound drainage blood. This blood is frequently reinfused unwashed and has been shown by several authors to contain a mixture of biologically active compounds, including activated complement.[11,12,43-47] Whereas some of these authors believe that the administration of recovered blood from wound drainage is safe, others contend that it is potentially risky with reports of hemodynamic instability, myocardial infarction, and hemostatic derangements. However, it is not clear whether these outcomes are the result of complement activation or of cytokine generation, fibrin degradation products, arachidonic acid metabolites, and other BRMs.

Influence of Leukocyte-Reduction Filters on Complement Activation

LR filters can enhance or diminish complement levels in plasma-containing blood components. Hetland et al[23] conducted a large study that analyzed complement activation with LR filters. The authors measured complement activation in pre- and postfiltration samples in five different red cell LR filters and four different platelet LR filters. Only two of the filters activated complement; the Imugard E red cell LR filter (Terumo Corp., Tokyo, Japan) and the Imugard IG500 platelet LR filter. The chemical composition of these filters differs substantially. The Imugard E is a polyvinyl alcohol adsorbent filter packed with polyethylene tetraphthalate and methylmethacrylate butadiene styrene copolymer. The Imugard IG500 filter is made of cotton wool. Holme et al[48] also demonstrated complement activation with the IG500 filter, whereas other studies showed complement activation with the Cellselect (NPBIbr, Emmer-Compaseum, The Netherlands), Sepacell PL5A (Asahi Medical Co., Tokyo, Japan), Sepacell R500A, and Pall RC50 (Pall Biomedical Products, Glen Cove, NY) LR filters.[22,49] The Cellselect is cellulose acetate, while the other filters are made with polyester fiber-based media. Because such a diversity of filter types can activate complement, a single mechanistic explanation for this activation is difficult to infer from a filter's chemical composition.

Because plasma contact with dialysis and other biologic filters has been known to activate complement it was presumed that some LR filters would do this too. However, recent data from several laboratories have shown that some LR filters can actually remove activated complement fragments. Ebert et al[50] demonstrated that greater than 80% of the anaphylatoxin C3a is removed from platelet concentrates with the PL100 polyester platelet LR filter. A similar scavenging ability was observed with the PL50 platelet LR filter,[22] the PXL-8 and PXL-A platelet LR filter, and the LPS plasma filter.[21,51] All of these filters are made with polyester fiber-based media.

Anaphylatoxins other than C3a are also selectively removed by some polyester fiber filters. One study showed the PL50 LR filter capable of removing greater than 90% of C4a from stored platelet concentrates or platelet-free plasma.[22] Measuring the removal of C5a is more difficult. Because of its potency, much smaller concentrations of C5a are biologically active.[27] The complement cascade frequently does not progress beyond C3 activation, and hence, when compared with C3a, smaller concentrations of C5a may be observed. Furthermore, C5a is tightly and rapidly bound to its receptor on leukocytes and may be bound to plastic component storage containers.[20,52] Therefore, little free C5a is seen in cellular blood components. In order to analyze C5a removal by LR filters, an in vitro system was established to augment levels of C5a in plasma. Plasma derived from Fresh Frozen Plasma (FFP) or platelet concentrates was treated with zymosan, a complement activator.[53] After removal of the zymosan by centrifugation, the plasma was filtered and aliquots of filtrate were tested for C5a. In this system, the PXL-8 and PXL-A platelet LR filters and the LPS plasma filter were indeed found capable of removing C5a from zymosan-treated plasma.[51]

Formation and Removal of Cytokines From Blood Components

While complement precursors are present in the acellular plasma fraction, cytokines are released from the cellular component in response to specific stimuli. Many cell types can secrete cytokines. The source of cytokines in stored blood components and recovered blood from wound drainage is, however, almost exclusively leukocytes. Activation of leukocytes promotes cytokine release (see Chapter 1). This activation may be the result of direct contact with bioincompatible surfaces or secondary to stimulation with activated complement, thrombin, or other cytokines and BRMs.

Cytokine accumulation is seen only in cellular blood products, such as granulocytes, whole blood, packed red blood cells, and platelet concentrates.[40,54-57] It is not seen in acellular products, such as FFP and cryoprecipitated antihemophiliac factor. When compared with red cell products, cytokine accumulation is particularly abundant in platelet concentrates. Whole blood or packed red blood cells are stored refrigerated, which decreases cellular metabolism and thus cytokine synthesis. In contrast, platelets are stored at room temperature. In studies by Stack et al,[54] the mean IL-8 concentration in units of packed red cells, conventionally stored for 42 days, was 512 ± 543 pg/mL. In contrast, conventionally stored units of random-donor platelet concentrates had a mean IL-8 concentration of 11,600 ± 31,300 pg/mL at only 5 days of storage.[55] Dramatic increases in levels of IL-1β, IL-6, TNFα, and RANTES with platelet concentrate storage have been observed in other studies.[7,21,40,56,58]

The physiologic impact of cytokines in blood components is poorly understood and difficult to study. Cytokines have widespread and diverse effects that frequently overlap. They are often involved in networks that influence both the formation of and the cellular responsiveness to other cytokines. Furthermore, only a limited number of cytokines have been analyzed in regard to transfusion. Nevertheless, there is now convincing evidence of a role for transfused cytokines, particularly IL-1β, IL-6, IL-8, and TNF-α in febrile nonhemolytic transfusion reactions. Some cytokines, such as IL-1β and TNF-α, probably cause fever by inducing prostaglandin E_2 synthesis in the hypothalamic thermoregulatory center.[59-61] Muylle et al[39] demonstrated an association of febrile nonhemolytic transfusion reactions with high levels of IL-6 and TNF-α. In a separate study, Muylle et al[62] showed a correlation between platelet concentrate storage time and probability of a febrile transfusion reaction. Presumably, this is the result of the increased accumulation of cytokines with increased storage time. Heddle et al[7] separated random-donor platelet concentrates into their plasma and cellular components. These were transfused into patients in random order with a 2-hour interval between transfusion. The probability of a febrile nonhemolytic reaction was more than three times greater with transfusion of the plasma component compared with the cellular component. Furthermore, a high level of plasma IL-1β and IL-6 correlated with the occurrence of a reaction.

The extent to which transfused cytokines are involved in other adverse reactions to blood components is not known. The levels of cytokines in some component units are indeed within the range shown to be clinically significant. For example, administration of 10-100 ng/kg of IL-1α or IL-1β has been shown to produce fever, anorexia, sleep, and a variety of acute-phase responses.[61] A dose of 5 μg/kg can induce hypotension. Stack et al[55] reported units of platelet concentrates with IL-1β concentrations greater than 2000 ng/L after 7 days of storage; Muylle et al[40] reported units with concentrations of IL-1β as high as 26,000 ng/L after 5 days of storage. If 300 mL of platelets with these IL-1 concentrations were infused into a 70-kg individual, they would correspond to infusions of 8.6 and 111 ng/kg of IL-1β respectively. As was seen for IL-1, other cytokines, such as IL-6 and TNF, may also be found at levels that would be expected to have a pharmacologic effect.[40,60,63]

Because cytokines in blood components are primarily produced by leukocytes, the most direct method to eliminate their production is to remove the offending leukocytes. Prestorage leukocyte reduction has been documented to be effective in preventing the accumulation of a variety of cytokines in stored blood components.[54,55,57] Unfortunately, prestorage leukocyte reduction is not always practical. It is costly, time-consuming, and, in some centers, logistically difficult.

In concept, poststorage leukocyte reduction should not be effective in removing cytokines from stored blood. To the contrary, leukocyte activation following binding to LR filter media would be expected to increase cytokine levels in the filtered component. However, limited data now show that poststorage leukocyte reduction can in fact reduce the quantity of some cytokines in the plasma of blood component. Both IL-8 and RANTES were selectively removed by the PXL-8 and PXL-A LR filters and the LPS plasma filter.[21,51] Although the efficiency of removing these substances was limited, it was possible to remove up to 97% of RANTES by sequential filtration of pooled platelet concentrates through four PXL-8 filters. In contrast, levels of IL-1β were not influenced by these LRFs.

Mechanisms for Removing Anaphylatoxins and Cytokines Through the Use of Biological Filters

Data showing that some polyester LR filters are capable of selectively removing the anaphylatoxins C3a, C4a, and C5a, and the cytokines IL-8 and RANTES suggest a new role for LR filters as BRM-scavenging devices. Maximizing the potential of these filters for this purpose requires an understanding of the mechanism for removal of these substances. While a detailed understanding is not currently available, potential mechanisms are suggested by available data on BRM filtration and current concepts of filter action.

One hypothesis is that leukocytes bound to the polyester fiber filters bind BRMs through their cell surface receptors. This is unlikely, as BRMs are as efficiently removed from acellular plasma as from cellular blood components. Alternatively, BRMs may bind directly to the filter media or to proteins bound to the filter media. These hypotheses have not been directly tested.

There is some evidence that electrostatic interactions are important for BRM filtration. Whereas the majority of circulating plasma proteins are anionic, those BRMs documented to be removed by polyester filters are cationic.[21,22,51] Thus, the pIs of IL-8, RANTES, C3a, and C5a are 8.0-8.5, 10.9, 8.6-9.6, and 8.6-9.6, respectively. In contrast, the BRMs shown to be unaffected by polyester filters, including IL-1β, IL-6, and TNF-α, are all neutral or acidic (pI = 6.8-7.0, 6.0-6.5, 5.6, respectively). Furthermore, acidification of filtered plasma inhibits the removal of RANTES by PXL-8 filters.[21] This may occur through the alteration of ionic interactions necessary for BRMs to bind to the filter. If cationic BRMs bind directly to the filter through ionic interactions, it is anticipated that they would be repulsed by and not attracted to LR filters with positively charged filter media. This indeed seems to be the case. The PLS-5A LR filter is similar to the PLS-10A filter that has been demonstrated to have a net-positive surface charge.[8] The PLS-5A LR filter is also unable to scavenge all cationic BRMs tested, including C3a, C5a, and IL-8 from plasma.[64]

If BRMs bind to filter media through simple noncovalent interactions, it is expected that a sufficient load of BRMs would saturate the LR filters. This may indeed be the case. Studies analyzing BRM concentration in sequential aliquots obtained during the course of filtration demonstrate that cytokine removal is dependent on filtration volume. For example, in one study, levels of IL-8 in the plasma filtrate reached a nadir with the PXL-8 filter after a 10-mL filtration volume and returned to prefiltration concentrations after 100 mL (Fig 3-2).[21] Similar findings were seen for filtrate levels of RANTES with the PXL-A filter, for IL-8 and RANTES with the LPS filter, and for C5a with the PXL-A, PXL-8, and LPS filters. Each level reached a nadir at a filtration volume of approximately 25 mL and then rose with continuing filtration.[51] These data support the concept that filter binding to BRMs is a saturable phenomenon. Once a filter's capacity is reached, additional BRMs are no longer removed.

The phenomenon of saturability may explain discrepant results on the removal of C3a by LR filters. Hetland et al[23] were unable to document removal of C3a with the PL-100 LR filter, but Ebert et al[50] demonstrated 81% removal. Shimuzu et al[22] demonstrated greater than 80% removal with the similar PL50 platelet LR filter. Shimuzu et al[22] attributed this discrepancy to

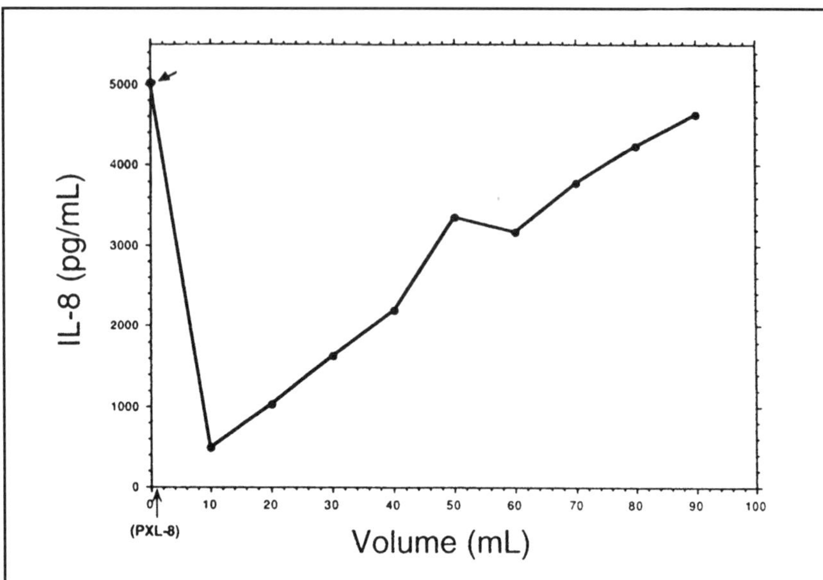

Figure 3-2. Single pilot study showing a reduction in IL-8 levels in postfiltration aliquots taken in every 10 mL after filtration through a PXL-8 filter. Results show an immediate marked decrease in IL-8 levels after filtration, with a slow increase back to baseline levels as filtration continues. The prefiltration level is indicated by a short arrow. (Used with permission from Snyder et al.[21])

methodologic differences. Hetland et al[23] used monoclonal antibodies to neoepitopes on activated C3 as an indirect measure of C3a, whereas Shimuzu et al[22] and Ebert et al[50] directly measured the C3a anaphylatoxin. Indeed, the neoepitopes measured may not have been adequately scavenged by the LR filters studied. However, it is also possible that the discrepancy in the results represents filter saturability. If the plasma concentration of C3 activation products in Hetland's study was high, even if some removal occurred, saturation may have been rapidly reached. Consequentially, the decrement in totally filtered C3a may not have been readily detected.

The data obtained so far are consistent with the idea that BRMs bind to filter media through simple, first-order kinetics governed by noncovalent interactions. It is also possible, however, that BRM removal is more complex. Binding of other proteins to solid surfaces has been shown to be complex. Kinetics of fibrinogen binding to glass surfaces is not first order. Rather, fibrinogen is initially taken up and then released after displacement by other plasma proteins.[65] This phenomenon is known as the Vroman effect. By analogy, the chemical environment of the filter is expected to change during the course of filtration. BRM removal is likely influenced by such environmental changes. Thus, the saturability observed in the removal of some BRMs may reflect the saturation of binding sites on the filter media. However, it is also possible that binding of other proteins creates an environment that prevents further BRM binding. Indeed, it is possible that, as for the Vroman effect, competitive displacement by other plasma proteins releases bound BRMs. Studies of the filtration of purified BRMs or BRMs admixed with known quantities of plasma proteins are required to discriminate between these possibilities.

Although the data are limited and definitive conclusions cannot be reached, analyses of BRM removal as a function of filtration volume suggest that different BRMs are not removed by a single mechanism. Thus, analysis of the efficiency of BRM removal as a function of filtration volume shows clear differences between individual BRMs. In one study by Snyder et al,[21] greater than 90% of RANTES in platelet-poor plasma is removed by the PXL-8 LR filter regardless of filtration volume. In contrast, at a 50-60 mL filtration volume removal of C3a was only 50% effective and by 75-85 mL only 30% effective. As the molar quantity of RANTES in the prefiltered material was greater than that of C3a; this is not simply a result of an overabundance of C3a saturating the filter. Rather, it seems that these two substances are not removed by a single mechanism. The mechanism responsible for C3a removal is more readily saturated than the mechanism responsible for RANTES removal. Similar results showing differences in the kinetics of BRM removal were observed in another study when filtration of IL-8, RANTES, C3a, and C5a were compared.[51]

All filters thus far documented that are capable of removing BRMs are composed of polyester fiber-based media. The processing of these media prior to their incorporation into filters is generally proprietary. Consequentially, it is not possible to know from the available data precisely how these filter media have been modified. An understanding of the properties of filter media that are important to BRM removal is necessary. Controlled studies analyzing media of defined composition will be important to eventually optimize filter design for BRM removal.

Generation of Bradykinin by Leukocyte-Reduction Filters

Bradykinin is a potent peptide capable of producing vasodilatation and shock.[66] Studies with dialysis membranes have shown contact-induced generation of bradykinin.[17] It is presumed that the negatively charged

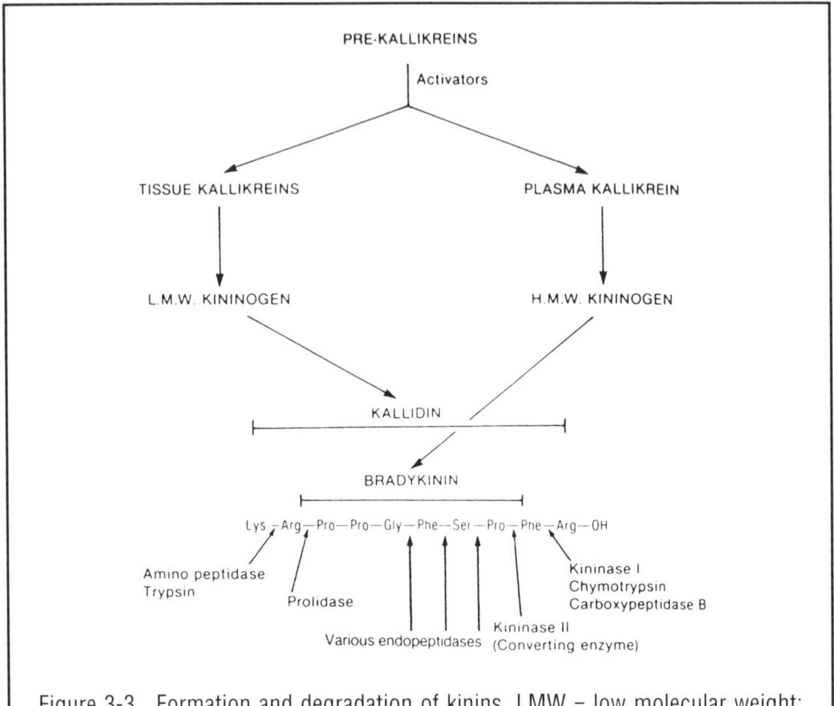

Figure 3-3 . Formation and degradation of kinins. LMW = low molecular weight; HMW = high molecular weight. (Used with permission from Regoli.[66])

membrane surface activates Factor XII of the intrinsic coagulation cascade (Fig 3-3).[67] The resulting Factor XIIa converts prekallikrein into kallikrein, which in turn catalyzes the formation of bradykinin from its precursor, high molecular weight kininogen.

The influence of bradykinin is extremely transient. It is degraded into smaller, biologically inactive peptides by two circulating enzymes: kininase I and kininase II. Angiotensin converting enzyme (ACE) is identical to kininase II. Because ACE inhibitors, such as captopril and enalapril, block the degradation of bradykinin, they can prolong the activity of bradykinin. Indeed, anaphylactoid reactions and hypotension attributable to bradykinin have been observed in patients receiving ACE inhibitors who then undergo hemodialysis or some apheresis procedures.[68-70]

Because many polyester LR filters are modified to enhance leukocyte trapping and because these modifications frequently result in a negatively charged filter medium, Takahashi et al[8,16] studied the impact of LR filters on bradykinin generation. Two platelet LR filters, the Pall PXL-8 and the Sepacell PLS-10A, were analyzed for surface charge. The PXL-8 was found to contain a negative charge and the PLS-10A a positive charge. Platelet concentrates were filtered through each of these devices. Little bradykinin was seen in prefiltration samples and in filtrates derived from the positively charged PLS-10A filter. In contrast, substantial amounts of bradykinin were observed after filtration with the negatively charged PXL-8 filter. The concentration of bradykinin in the filtrate was approximately 10-fold greater in an aliquot removed half way through the filtration compared with an aliquot removed at the completion of filtration. This was interpreted to imply that the bradykinin formed because of contact activation on the filter surface is actively degraded by kininases in the filtrate after filtration. This contention is further supported by the observation that the addition of ACE inhibitors to the platelet concentrates not only increases the peak levels of bradykinin but also preserves that peak level through the course of filtration.[16] Krailadsiri and Seghatchian[15] similarly observed that platelet concentrates filtered through the negatively charged Pall PL50D LR filter had increased kallikrein-like activity. Interestingly, Factor XII activity was not increased, suggesting that the normal route of contact activation is bypassed or that the Factor XIIa is not detectable because it binds to surfaces or inhibitors.

It is not known whether bradykinin formed as a result of transfusing plasma-based components through LR filters is clinically harmful. There is evidence to suggest that it is. Cases of anaphylactoid hypotension have been described in patients receiving leukocyte-reduced platelet concentrates at the bedside.[71] Sano et al[72] described a 12-year-old female with aplastic anemia and chronic renal failure who repeatedly developed hypotension in response to the administration of irradiated platelet concentrates through a negatively charged (Pall PL-50D) LR filter. These episodes responded rapidly to discontinuation of the infusion but did not respond to antihistamines. Upon switching to a positively charged filter (Sepacell PLS-5A), no further reactions were seen. Although the authors do not state whether the patient was receiving ACE inhibitors, the history is suggestive of a bradykinin-induced reaction.

Fried et al[73] similarly reported a patient who consistently had hypotensive reactions when receiving FFP that was administered with a single LR filter type (Pall RC XL1C). Prior transfusion of FFP through a different, positively charged filter (Sepacell PLS-5A) and subsequent transfusions without LR filters were uneventful.

Formation and Removal of Histamine and Other Biological Response Modifiers

Histamine is a vasoactive amino acid with a variety of physiologic effects, including increased capillary permeability, hypotension, and bronchoconstriction. These effects resemble those seen in anaphylactoid-type transfusion reactions. Frewin et al[74] studied a cohort of patients experiencing anaphylactoid reactions and found significantly elevated plasma histamine levels. This elevation was not seen in patients having febrile reactions, mixed-type reactions, or no reaction.

Histamine accumulates in blood components at a rate dependent on leukocyte content.[75] Leukocyte reduction by prestorage filtration effectively prevents the accumulation of histamine by removing the source leukocytes.[76,77] The clinical impact of histamine transfused with blood components is not known. Plasma levels of approximately 1 ng/mL have been reported in patients experiencing anaphylactoid symptoms.[74,78] Platelet concentrates with levels as high as 22 ng/mL (1100 ng/50 mL platelet concentrate) have been reported.[74] Although the half-life of circulating histamine is brief, rapid infusion of multiple units containing equivalently large histamine loads is anticipated to have physiologic consequences. This is further suggested by data showing that patients who have anaphylactoid transfusion reactions are likely to have received more and older units of blood components compared with those not having these reactions.[73] Definitive proof that this increased susceptibility to anaphylactoid reactions is the result of infusion of histamine, however, is lacking. Such evidence is difficult to acquire because of the episodic and currently unpredictable nature of anaphylactoid reactions, the presence of multiple concurrent factors that may influence susceptibility, and the impact of other vasoactive BRMs, such as serotonin, that may influence these reactions.

Various other BRMs have been observed in the plasma of stored blood components. These include fibrin degradation products, β-thromboglobulin, and platelet factor 4. Although some of these substances are suspected of playing a role in the platelet storage lesion, it is not known whether they have any adverse clinical effect on transfusion. Interestingly, one study failed to show an effect of the PL-50 poststorage LR filter on β-thromboglobulin and platelet factor 4.[22] The influence of prestorage LR filters on the levels of these substances is not known.

Conclusions

Increasing evidence supports a role for BRMs in adverse reactions to transfused blood components. These BRMs include cytokines, activated complement, vasoactive peptides, and amino acids. They form primarily as a consequence of the bioincompatability of materials used for collecting, storing, and processing blood as well as secondary activation of leukocytes and platelets. Because histamine and most of the cytokines are produced by leukocytes, their accumulation can be minimized by prestorage leukocyte reduction. However, prestorage leukocyte reduction cannot prevent the generation of activated complement, bradykinin, or other plasma-derived BRMs.

Recent data demonstrate that several poststorage polyester LR filters are capable of removing the anaphylatoxins C3a, C4a, and C5a, and the cytokines IL-8 and RANTES from plasma-containing blood components. The mechanism of this removal is not known but may involve electrostatic interactions between BRMs and the filter. Because these filters were designed only for effective leukocyte removal, they have not been optimized for BRM removal. The clinical significance of the limited abilities of the current generation of filters to remove BRMs is uncertain. However, a better understanding of the mechanisms of BRM removal may lead to the improved bioengineering of filters. Filters with large binding capacities for BRMs may eventually prove clinically useful. Such filters not only may improve transfusion practice by decreasing the incidence and severity of reactions due to transfused BRMs, but also may find use in other applications where BRMs mediate disease. In-line BRM filters may eventually prove helpful in cardiopulmonary bypass, reinfusion of recovered blood from wound drainage, sepsis, multiorgan failure, and a variety of other conditions. Clearly, our understanding of the potential of filtration as a means of altering the content of BRMs in plasma has not been realized. Further study of this topic will likely lead to even safer transfusion practice and the development of new therapies for BRM-mediated disease.

References

1. Demling R. The modern version of adult respiratory distress syndrome. Ann Rev Med 1995;46:193-202.
2. St. John R, Dorinsky P. Immunologic therapy for ARDS, septic shock, and multi-organ failure. Chest 1993;103:932-43.

3. Espat N, Moldawer L, Copeland E. Cytokine-mediated alterations in host metabolism prevent nutritional repletion in cachetic cancer patients. J Surg Oncol 1995;58:77-82.
4. Zumkeller W, Schofield P. Growth factors, cytokines, and soluble forms of receptor molecules in cancer patients. Anticancer Res 1995;15:344-8.
5. Cavallo M, Pozzilli P, Thorpe R. Cytokines and autoimmunity. Clin Exp Immunol 1994;96:1-7.
6. Gianani R, Sarvetnick N. Viruses, cytokines, antigens, and autoimmunity. Proc Natl Acad Sci USA 1996;93:2257-9.
7. Heddle N, Klama L, Singer J, et al. The role of plasma from platelet concentrates in transfusion reactions. N Engl J Med 1994;331:625-8.
8. Takahashi T, Abe H, Hosoda M, et al. Bradykinin generation during filtration of platelet concentrates with a white cell reduction filter (letter). Transfusion 1995;35:967.
9. Rinder C, Rinder H, Smith B, et al. Blockade of C5a and C5b-9 generation inhibits leukocyte and platelet activation during extracorporeal circulation. J Clin Invest 1995;96:1564-72.
10. Rinder C, Bohnert J, Rinder H, et al. Platelet activation and aggregation during cardiopulmonary bypass. Anesthesiology 1991;75:388-93.
11. Clements DH, Sculco TP, Burke SW, et al. Salvage and reinfusion of postoperative sanguineous wound drainage: A preliminary report. J Bone Joint Surg Am 1992;74:646-51.
12. Southern E, Huo M, Mehta J, Keggi K. Unwashed wound drainage blood. What are we giving our patients? Clin Orthop 1995;320:235-46.
13. Busund R, Balteskard L, Ronning G, et al. Fatal myocardial depression and circulatory collapse associated with complement activation induced by plasma infusion in severe porcine sepsis. Acta Anaesthesiol Scand 1995;39:100-8.
14. Finn A, Naik S, Klein N, et al. Interleukin-8 release and neutrophil degranulation after pediatric cardiopulmonary bypass. J Thorac Cardiovasc Surg 1993;105:234-41.
15. Krailadsiri P, Seghatchian J. Negatively charged leukocyte filter significantly enhances kallikrein and thrombin-like activities of platelet concentrates. Thromb Res 1996;83:469-74.
16. Takahashi T, Abe H, Fujihara M, et al. Quality of platelet components: The role of suspension medium and complement depletion. Transfus Clin Biol 1994;6:481-7.

17. Ahmad S. Hemodialysis. Curr Nephrol 1996;327-63.
18. Janatova J, Cheung A, Parker C. Biomedical polymers differ in their capacity to activate complement. Complement Inflamm 1991;8:61-9.
19. Gawaz M, Bogner C. Changes in platelet membrane glycoproteins and platelet leukocyte interactions during hemodialysis. Clin Investig 1994;72:424-9.
20. Gyongyossy-Issa MI, McLeod EL, Devine D. Complement activation in platelet concentrates is surface-dependent and modulated by the platelets. J Lab Clin Med 1994;123:859-68.
21. Snyder E, Mechanic S, Baril L, Davenport R. Removal of soluble biological response modifiers (complement and chemokines) by a bedside leukoreduction filter. Transfusion 1996;36:707-13.
22. Shimizu T, Uchigiri C, Mizuno S, et al. Adsorption of anaphylatoxins and platelet-specific proteins by filtration of platelet concentrates with a polyester leukocyte-reduction filter. Vox Sang 1994;66:161-5.
23. Hetland G, Mollnes T, Larsen J, Garred P. Biocompatibility of white cell filters as evaluated by complement activation. Transfusion 1992;32:557-61.
24. Bruil A, Buegeling T, Feijen J, Aken WV. The mechanisms of leukocyte removal by filtration. Transfus Med Rev 1995;9:145-66.
25. Lane T. Leukocyte reduction of cellular blood components. Arch Pathol Lab Med 1994;118:392-404.
26. Sims P, Wiedmer T. Complement biology. 2nd ed. In: Hoffman EA, ed. Hematology. New York: Churchill Livingstone, 1995:154-6.
27. Hugli T. Bioactive factors of the blood complement system. In: Bradshaw RA, ed. Proteins in biology and medicine. New York: Academic Press 1982:91-116.
28. Sims PJ. Interaction of human platelets with the complement system. In: Kunick TJ, George JN, eds. Platelet immunology. Philadelphia: Lippincott-Raven, 1989:354.
29. Polley M, Nachman R. Human platelet activation by C3a and C3a des-arg. J Exp Med 1983:158:603-15.
30. Haeffner-Cavaillon N, Cavaillon JM, Laude M, Kazatchkine M. C3a(C3a des-arg) induces production and release of interleukin 1 by cultured human monocytes. J Immunol 1987;139:794-9.
31. Chenoweth D, Cooper S, Hugli T, et al. Complement activation during cardiopulmonary bypass. N Engl J Med 1981;304:497-503.
32. Craddock P, Fehr J, Dalmasso A, et al. Hemodialysis leukopenia: Pulmonary vascular leukostasis resulting from complement activation by dialyzer cellophane membranes. J Clin Invest 1977;59:879-88.

33. Mollison PL, Engelfriet CP, Contreras M. The withdrawal of blood. In: Blood transfusion in clinical medicine. 9th ed. Oxford: Blackwell Scientific, 1993:2-47.
34. Schleuning M, Bock M, Mempel W. Complement activation during storage of single donor platelet concentrates. Vox Sang 1994;67:144-8.
35. Miletic V, Popovic O. Complement activation in stored platelet concentrates. Transfusion 1993;33:150-4.
36. Larsson A, Egberg N, Lindahl T. Platelet activation and binding of complement components to platelets induced by immune complexes. Platelets 1994;5:149-55.
37. Bode A, Miller D. Generation and degradation of fibrinopeptide A in stored platelet concentrate. Vox Sang 1986;51:192-6.
38. Wiedmer T, Esmon C, Sims P. Complement proteins C5b-9 stimulate procoagulant activity through platelet prothrombinase. Blood 1986; 68:875-80.
39. Sims P, Faioni E, Wiedmer T, Shattil S. Complement proteins C5b-9 cause release of membrane vesicles from the platelet surface that are enriched in the membrane receptor for coagulation factor Va and express prothrombinase activity. J Biol Chem 1988;263:18205-12.
40. Muylle L, Joos M, Wouters E, et al. Increased tumor necrosis factor α, (TNF-alpha), interleukin 1 (IL-1), and interleukin 6 (IL-6) levels in the plasma of stored platelet concentrates: Relationship between TNF α and IL-6 levels and febrile transfusion reactions. Transfusion 1993;33: 195-9.
41. Evans R, Turner E, Bingham M. Studies with radioiodinated cold agglutinins of ten patients. Am J Med 1965;38:378-95.
42. Sherman S, Taswell H. The need for transfusion of saline washed red blood cells to patients with paroxysmal nocturnal hemoglobinuria: A myth. Transfusion 1977;17:683.
43. Bengston J, Backman L, Stenqvist O, et al. Complement activation and reinfusion of wound drainage blood. Anesthesiology 1990;73: 376-80.
44. Blevins FT, Shaw B, Valeri CR, et al. Reinfusion of shed blood after orthopaedic procedures in children and adolescents. J Bone Joint Surg 1993;75:363-71.
45. Healy WL, Pfeiffer BA, Kurtz SR, et al. Evaluation of autologous shed blood for autotransfusion after orthopaedic surgery. Clin Orthop 1994;299:53-9.
46. Schonberger J, Oeveren WV, Bredee J, et al. Systemic blood activation during and after autotransfusion. Ann Thorac Surg 1994;57:1256-62.

47. Sieunarine K, Lawrence-Brown M, Brennan E, et al. The quality of blood used for transfusion. J Cardiovasc Surg 1992;33:98-105.
48. Holme S, Ross D, Heaton W. in vitro and in vivo evaluation of platelet concentrates after cotton wool filtration. Vox Sang 1989;57:112-5.
49. Gu Y, Obster R, Haan J, et al. Biocompatibility of leukocyte removal filters during leukocyte filtration of cardiopulmonary bypass perfusate. Artif Organs 1993;17:660-5.
50. Ebert S, Britt C, Reddy R, et al. Safety and efficacy of a new platelet white cell removal filter (abstract). Transfusion 1989;29:10S.
51. Geiger T, Baril L, Dincecco D, et al. Selective removal of anaphylatoxin C3a and C5a and chemokines IL-8 and RANTES by bedside polyester-fiber leukodepletion and plasma filters (abstract). Blood 1996;88S1:530a.
52. Oppermann M, Gotze O. Plasma clearance of human C5a anaphylatoxin by binding to leukocyte C5a receptors. Immunology 1994; 82:516-21.
53. Marcus-Bagley D, Alper C. Methods for allotyping complement proteins. In: Rose N, ed. Manual of clinical laboratory immunology. 4th ed. Washington, DC: American Society for Microbiology, 1992:124-41.
54. Stack G, Baril L, Napychank P, Snyder E. Cytokine generation in stored, white cell reduced, and bacterially contaminated units of red cells. Transfusion 1995;35:199-203.
55. Stack G, Snyder E. Cytokine generation in stored platelet concentrates. Transfusion 1994;34:20-5.
56. Bubel S, Wilhelm D, Entelman M, et al. Chemokines in stored platelet concentrates. Transfusion 1996;36:445-9.
57. Flegel W, Wiesneth M, Stampe D, Koerner K. Low cytokine contamination in buffy coat derived platelet concentrates without filtration. Transfusion 1995;35:917-20.
58. Aye M, Palmer D, Giulivi A, Hashemi S. Effect of filtration of platelet concentrates on the accumulation of cytokines and platelet release factors during storage. Transfusion 1995;35:117-25.
59. Rosendorff C, Mooney J. Central nervous system sites of action of a purified leukocyte pyrogen. Am J Physiol 1971;220:597-603.
60. Chapman P, Lester T, Casper E, et al. Clinical pharmacology of recombinant human tumor necrosis factor in patients with advanced cancer. J Clin Oncol 1987;5:1942-51.
61. Dinarello C. Interleukin-1 and interleukin-1 antagonism. Blood 1991; 77:1627-52.

62. Muylle L, Wouters E, De Bock R, Peetermans ME. Reactions to platelet transfusion: The effect of the storage time of the concentrate. Transfus Med 1992;2:289-93.
63. Nijsten MW, De Groot ER, Ten Duis HJ, et al. Serum levels of interleukin-6 and acute phase responses (letter). Lancet 1987;2:921.
64. Geiger T, Snyder EL. Removal of anaphylatoxins C3a and C5a and chemokines Il-8 and RANTES by polyester leukoreduction filters. Transfusion 1997;37(in press).
65. Vroman L, Adams A, Fischer G, Munoz P. Interaction of high molecular weight kininogen, factor XII, and fibrinogen in plasma at interfaces. Blood 1980;55:156-9.
66. Wachtfogel Y, Cadena RD, Colman R. Structural biology, cellular interactions, and pathophysiology of the contact system. Thromb Res 1993;72:1-23.
67. Regoli D. Polypeptides et antagonistes. In: Firoud JP, Mathé G, Meyniel G, eds. Pharmacologie clinique: Bases de la thérapeutique. 2nd ed. Paris: Expansion Scientifique Francaise, 1988:691.
68. Olbricht C, Schaumann D, Fischer D. Anaphylactoid reactions, LDL apheresis with dextran sulfate, and ACE inhibitors. Lancet 1992;340: 908-9.
69. Davidson D, Peart I, Turner S, Sangster M. Prevention with icatibant of anaphylactoid reactions to ACE inhibitor during LDL apheresis (letter). Lancet 1994;343:1575.
70. Verresen L, Waer M, Vanrenterghem Y, Michielsen P. Angiotensin converting enzyme inhibitors and anaphylactoid reactions to high flux membrane dialysis. Lancet 1990;336:1360-2.
71. Hume H, Popovsky M, Benson K, et al. Hypotensive reactions: A previously uncharacterized complication of platelet transfusion? Transfusion 1996;36:904-9.
72. Sano H, Koga Y, Hamasaki K, et al. Anaphylaxis associated with white-cell reduction filter (letter). Lancet 1996;347:1053.
73. Fried MR, Eastlund T, Christie B, et al. Hypotensive reactions to white cell-reduced plasma in a patient undergoing angiotensin-converting enzyme inhibitor therapy. Transfusion 1996;36:900-3.
74. Frewin D, Jonsson J, Russell W, et al. Influence of blood storage time and plasma histamine levels on the pattern of transfusion reactions. Vox Sang 1989;56:243-6.
75. Muylle L, Lekeman G, Herman AG, Peetermans ME. Histamine levels in stored platelet concentrates: Relationship to white cell content. Transfusion 1988;28:226-8.

76. Frewin D, Jonsson J, Davis K, et al. Effect of microfiltration on the histamine levels in stored human blood. Vox Sang 1987;52:191-4.
77. Frewin DB, Dyer SM, Haylock DN, et al. A comparative study of the effect of three methods of leukocyte removal on plasma histamine levels in stored human blood. Semin Hematol 1991;28S5:18-21.
78. Ind P, Barnes P, Brown M, et al. Measurement of plasma histamine in asthma. Clin Allergy 1983;13:61-7.

In: Davenport RD, Snyder EL, eds.
Cytokines in Transfusion Medicine: A Primer
Bethesda, MD: AABB Press, 1997

4

Inflammatory Cytokines in Hemolytic Transfusion Reactions

ROBERTSON D. DAVENPORT, MD

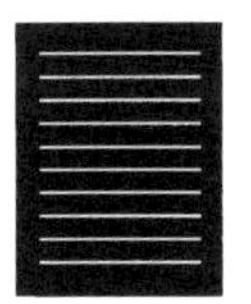

HEMOLYTIC TRANSFUSION REACTIONS (HTRs) HAVE long been recognized as a paradigm of the systemic inflammatory response. Classically, HTRs present a spectrum of signs and symptoms that include fever, rigors, hypotension, renal failure, respiratory failure, intravascular coagulation, and possibly death. There is clearly a close clinical similarity between HTRs and sepsis in which the pathophysiologic role of cytokines is now established. While the involvement of activation products in the classical pathway of complement in the pathophysiology of HTRs has been established, there is an increasing body of evidence indicating that cytokines have a central role in these reactions.

Robertson D. Davenport, MD, Assistant Professor of Pathology, University of Michigan Medical School, Ann Arbor, Michigan

Immune hemolysis stimulates the production of several cytokines that are likely to prove crucial to the initiation, maintenance, and ultimate resolution of HTRs (Table 4-1)[1]. The biology of cytokines is reviewed in Chapter 1. There is strong evidence for the participation of at least three categories of cytokines in HTRs: proinflammatory cytokines, chemokines, and anti-inflammatory cytokines.

Table 4-1. Cytokines Implicated in Hemolytic Transfusion Reactions[1]

Terminology	Biologic Activities
Proinflammatory Cytokines: IL-1 TNF	Fever Hypotension, shock, death (synergy) Mobilization of leukocytes from marrow Activation of T and B cells Induction of cytokines (IL-1, IL-6, IL-8, TNF, MCP-1) Induction of adhesion molecules Induction of procoagulants
IL-6	Fever Acute phase protein response B-cell antibody production T-cell activation
Chemokines: IL-8	Chemotaxis of neutrophils Chemotaxis of lymphocytes Neutrophil activation Basophil histamine release
MCP-1	Chemotaxis of monocytes Induction of respiratory burst Induction of adhesion molecules Induction of IL-1
Anti-inflammatory cytokines: IL-1ra	Competitive inhibition of IL-1 type I and II receptors

IL-1 = interleukin-1; TNF = tumor necrosis factor; IL-6 = interleukin-6; IL-8 = interleukin-8; MCP-1 = monocyte chemoattractant protein-1; IL-1ra = interleukin-1 receptor antagonist. (Used with permission from Davenport.[1])

Proinflammatory Cytokines

The proinflammatory cytokines, tumor necrosis factor (TNF), interleukin-1 (IL-1), and interleukin-6 (IL-6) are pyrogens. The production of these mediators during immune hemolysis is responsible for the clinical hallmarks of fever and rigors. These cytokines also activate a number of cell types to produce other cytokines, express leukocyte adhesion receptor molecules, and promote procoagulant activity.

Leukocytosis, with an absolute granulocytosis, often accompanies HTRs. This may be particularly evident in extravascular hemolysis of delayed HTRs in which fever and neutrophilia can suggest the presence of occult infection. Chemokines that are produced during immune hemolysis, particularly interleukin-8 (IL-8), recruit leukocytes from marrow. These mediators are directly responsible for the observed leukocytosis. Indirectly, other cytokines, such as IL-1, also stimulate hematopoiesis.

Intravascular coagulation is also a recognized complication of HTRs, particularly those involving complement-fixing red cell antibodies such as within the ABO system. The proinflammatory cytokines IL-1 and TNF have been shown to promote coagulation by several mechanisms that include the expression of tissue factor by monocytes and endothelial cells and the down-regulation of endothelial cell surface thrombomodulin. Several other mechanisms for the initiation of disseminated intravascular coagulation (DIC) in this setting have been proposed, such as the activation of platelets by circulating immune complexes, the activation of the contact system of coagulation by consumption of the major inhibitor C1-esterase inhibitor, and the liberation of thromboplastic substances from lysed red cells. However, there is relatively little experimental data to support these conjectures.

Hemolytic transfusion reactions are also associated with the production of new allo- and autoantibodies as well as augmentation in the strength of preexisting red cell antibodies. Antibody production requires the coordinated actions of antigen-presenting cells, T lymphocytes, and B lymphocytes. It is now clear that this process is coordinated by several cytokines, including IL-1 and IL-6, that may be produced during immune hemolysis. IL-1 is a cofactor for T-cell activation and augments B-cell proliferation and differentiation. IL-6 enhances antibody production by committed B lymphocytes; thus, systemic production of these mediators during HTRs promotes red cell antibody responses.

Proinflammatory Cytokine Production in ABO Incompatibility

Evidence that TNF production is strongly stimulated by ABO incompatibility comes from both in-vitro experiments and clinical observations. Using a whole blood model of ABO incompatibility in which allogeneic red blood cells (RBCs) are incubated with fresh heparinized whole blood, TNF is produced in a dose- and time-dependent manner when incompatible RBCs are added.[2] However, when compatible (group O) RBCs are added, no TNF production is detectable. The addition of group A, B, or AB RBCs causes TNF production that is indistinguishable among each of these three conditions. Incubation of RBCs in plasma that is devoid of leukocytes results in hemolysis of incompatible RBCs, as expected, without TNF production.

TNF is an early-response cytokine that appears in plasma within 2 hours of stimulation by incompatible RBCs and remains at peak levels for approximately 2 hours. Thereafter, plasma TNF levels decline and are similar to unstimulated control samples at 24 hours. The regulation of TNF production in whole blood in response to ABO incompatibility appears to be at the level of gene transcription similar to other well-characterized stimuli, such as endotoxin. TNF gene expression by peripheral blood leukocytes is strongly stimulated by ABO-incompatible RBCs and is superinducible by the addition of the protein synthesis inhibitor cycloheximide. This indicates that TNF gene expression in this setting is most likely under the regulation of short-lived repressor proteins. Active complement is required for TNF expression in response to ABO incompatibility. In vitro experiments have shown that when complement is inactivated, neither hemolysis of incompatible red cells nor significant TNF production occurs.

Production of TNF has also been demonstrated in vivo during a hemolytic transfusion reaction, in a group O patient who inadvertently received 100 mL of group A RBCs.[3] This patient was on a protocol in which TNF levels and neutrophil elastase were measured as part of a study of physiologic responses to cardiopulmonary bypass.[4] Both of these became elevated after the patient received the incompatible blood transfusion. The time for TNF to appear in plasma was similar to that observed in vitro. The release of neutrophil elastase in this patient increased progressively over 24 hours as expected if IL-8, which can induce neutrophil degranulation, was produced in response to the incompatible transfusion (see below). Since no other patient in this protocol showed a significant rise in plasma TNF levels during surgery, the cytokine response was certainly due to the incompatible transfusion.

Proinflammatory Cytokine Production in Extravascular Hemolysis

The proinflammatory cytokines IL-1β, IL-6, and TNF are also produced in IgG-mediated extravascular hemolysis.[5,6] The production time and relative quantity of these proteins produced differ from the setting of ABO incompatibility. IL-1β and IL-6 appear in response to IgG-coated red cells progressively over at least 24 hours. In contrast, TNF is produced in a somewhat delayed fashion in that it is not significantly elevated except at 6 hours. However, cell-associated TNF can be demonstrated by immunocytochemical staining in monocytes engaged in erythrophagocytosis.

There appear to be two categories of cytokine responses in the setting of extravascular hemolysis: those produced at high levels greater than 1 ng/mL by 24 hours and others produced at lower levels in the range of 100 pg/mL.[5] Low-level cytokine responses include IL-1β, IL-6, and TNF. IL-8 is a high-level response cytokine that is produced on a time course similar to its production in the setting of ABO incompatibility. In contrast, TNF is produced in a delayed fashion in response to IgG-coated red cells, achieving a level of less than 100 pg/mL.

In summary, while the in-vitro models employed in studies of ABO and IgG-mediated red cell incompatibility are not directly comparable, these findings do suggest a possible reason for the clinical differences between intravascular and extravascular HTRs. In the former case, TNF is released into systemic circulation where it can have diverse effects on many cell types; whereas, in the latter case, TNF effects may be confined to local effects at the site of erythrophagocytosis, primarily the spleen.

Chemokine Production in ABO Incompatibility

The chemokines interleukin-8 (IL-8) and monocyte chemoattractant protein-1 (MCP-1) are strongly stimulated by ABO incompatibility.[7,8] These chemokines are produced on a different time course than that of TNF. There is a delay of 4-6 hours following stimulation before these chemokines are detectable in plasma. Thereafter, these chemokines are produced progressively over at least 24 hours and reach very high levels in plasma. As is the case with TNF, gene expression for these chemokines is strongly stimulated by ABO incompatibility. Active complement is also required for their expression in whole blood.

Chemokine Production in Extravascular Hemolysis

There is a strong similarity between ABO- and IgG-mediated incompatibility models in the production of IL-8 and MCP-1. These chemokines are produced on similar time courses and in comparable quantities in both settings. There are differences, however, in the regulation of these cellular responses. In IgG-mediated incompatibility, cytokine production appears to be largely the result of interactions between the IgG receptor FcγRI and the red-cell-bound IgG. In this setting cytokine production can be inhibited by soluble human IgG but not by Fab fragments of monoclonal antibody IV.3, which is specific for the second major class of human IgG receptors present on monocytes FcγRII. This correlates with evidence that erythrophagocytosis by monocytes is mediated by FcγRI.[9] This dependence on high-affinity IgG receptors explains why it is so unusual to see erythrophagocytosis on peripheral blood smears from patients with delayed HTRs or autoimmune hemolytic anemia resulting from IgG antibodies that do not fix complement, despite large numbers of IgG-coated red cells in circulation. When immunoglobulins are at normal levels in circulation, the monocyte FcγRI is occupied by nonspecific monomeric IgG and, thus, unavailable to red-cell-bound IgG.[10] The role of the third major class of IgG receptors, FcγRIII, in HTRs is under investigation. This receptor is not present on peripheral blood monocytes but is strongly expressed on macrophages, including those of the spleen.[11] FcγRIII may have a major role in the clearance of IgG-coated red cells and platelets in autoimmune hemolytic anemia and autoimmune thrombocytopenia, where there is evidence that a blockade of FcγRIII by a specific monoclonal antibody, 3G8, will ameliorate these diseases.[12,13] Furthermore, alloantibodies mediate the binding of red cells to splenic macrophages in vitro through FcγRIII.[14]

Anti-Inflammatory Cytokine Production in Extravascular Hemolysis

IgG-mediated hemolysis also strongly stimulates the production of the IL-1 inhibitor IL-1ra.[15] Significant levels of IL-1ra appear in a parallel fashion to IL-1β. Immunocytochemical staining has demonstrated strong reactivity to IL-1ra in monocytes engaged in erythrophagocytosis. Northern blot analysis of mononuclear cell ribonucleic acid (RNA) shows that IL-1 gene expression precedes that of IL-1ra in response to IgG-coated red cells. However, neutralizing antibodies to IL-1 do not suppress either IL-1ra or IL-1β gene expression in response to IgG-coated red cells. Therefore, it appears that IL-1ra production is a primary response to erythrophagocytosis rather than an autocrine phenomenon induced by initial IL-1 production. It is interesting that dexamethasone inhibits both IL-1 and IL-1ra production by monocytes in response to IgG-coated red cells. These data suggest the possibility that the clinical variability of delayed HTRs and some of the clinical differences from intravascular HTRs may be accounted for, in part, by the relative balance of IL-1 and IL-1ra production.

Target Cells of Cytokines Produced During Red Cell Incompatibility

The biologic mediators produced during HTRs affect many cell types. One cell that is closely involved in these reactions is the endothelial cell. Since the endothelium lines the entire vasculature, cytokines in systemic circulation have immediate access to these cells. Under normal circumstances, the endothelium provides a semipermeable barrier and an anticoagulant surface that are essential to maintaining the microenvironment of circulation. However, under the influences of the proinflammatory cytokines IL-1 and TNF, endothelial cells will express leukocyte adhesion receptors and chemotactic factors and will alter their surface characteristics to favor thrombosis. The substantial levels of TNF that are produced in whole blood in response to ABO-incompatible red cells can induce these responses in the endothelium.

When cultured human umbilical vein endothelial cells are stimulated with conditioned plasma derived from whole blood incubated with ABO-incompatible red cells, the endothelial cells express the leukocyte adhesion molecules intercellular adhesion molecule-1 (ICAM-1) and E-selectin (also termed endothelial-leukocyte adhesion molecule-1 or ELAM-1) (unpublished data.) In addition, these cells elaborate the leukocyte chemotactic factors IL-8 and MCP-1 under the same stimuli. Northern blot analysis of endothelial cell mRNA indicates that gene expression for ICAM-1, ELAM-1, IL-8, and MCP-1 are all strongly induced by the conditioned plasma for ABO-incompatibility reactions. Control plasma from whole blood incubated with compatible red cells does not induce gene expression or protein production for any of these molecules. The addition of neutralizing anti-TNF to the conditioned plasma at the time of endothelial cell stimulation completely abrogates the production of both adhesion molecules and chemotactic factors by the endothelial cells. Thus, the necessary conditions for leukocyte infiltration of tissues are established in these reactions as a direct consequence of TNF production.

Furthermore, endothelial cells incubated with conditioned plasma from ABO incompatibility reactions produce a procoagulant that initiates clotting through a Factor VII-dependent mechanism (unpublished data). This procoagulant activity can be blocked by specific antibodies to tissue factor. Analysis of tissue factor mRNA expression by quantitative polymerase chain reaction technique shows that gene expression is increased approximately 100-fold in response to conditioned plasma. Similarly to the case with adhesion molecule and cytokine induction, neutralized anti-TNF added to the stimulating medium prevents the induction of this procoagulant activity.

Implications of Cytokine Responses in Hemolytic Transfusion Reactions

Proinflammatory Cytokines

The proinflammatory cytokines TNF, IL-1, and IL-6 appear to be the principal causes of fever, the activation of leukocytes, and the stimulation of procoagulant activity during an HTR. IL-1 and TNF share many common features, although they are the products of distinct genes. Since each of these cytokines will induce the gene expression of the other, they can be thought of as two sides of the same coin with regard to their roles in HTRs. An important biologic activity of IL-1 and TNF is that, at sufficient concentrations in blood, they both will cause circulatory collapse, shock, and death. Furthermore, IL-1 and TNF exert a synergistic effect in this respect.[16]

IL-1 and TNF have a complex effect on leukocytes that results in activation and promotes antibody responses. IL-1 will stimulate hematopoiesis and is involved in the recruitment and activation of neutrophils from the marrow. This effect may be mediated through the induction of chemokines such as IL-8. IL-1 is also involved in cellular and humoral immune responses at several levels. Lymphocyte activation is a complex process that involves antigen presentation and accessory signals, which in part is dependent on IL-1. IL-1 potentiates the proliferative response of splenic B cells to mitogenic stimuli[16]; enhances the generation of immunoglobulin-secreting cells from B cells in response to T-cell-derived signals[17]; and increases the number of activated cells, cell cycle progression, and IL-2 production by mitogen-stimulated T cells.[18]

IL-6 is involved in several stages of B-cell development in that it stimulates both proliferation and differentiation. Antibody production by differentiated B cells is enhanced by the addition of IL-6 and markedly reduced by neutralizing antibodies to IL-6.[19] IL-6 plays a role in responses to red cell antigens since both primary and secondary antibody responses to sheep red cells by mice are significantly enhanced by IL-6, both in vivo and in vitro.[20] IL-6 is necessary for the growth of many hybridoma cell lines, a fact that has been used for bioassays.[21] The actions of IL-6 on T cells are not as well characterized as those on B cells. However, it is clear that IL-6 will stimulate the proliferation of mature T cells in concert with T-cell receptor ligation and can largely replace the function of mononuclear phagocytes as an accessory signal for T-cell activation.[22,23] IL-1 potentiates this response, not only by inducing IL-6 production, but also by increasing the responsiveness of T cells to IL-6.[24,25]

Chemokines

Chemokines, the second class of cytokines involved in HTRs, are produced primarily by mononuclear phagocytes, in a similar manner to the pro-inflammatory cytokines, but have a much more restricted range of target cells. Chemokines usually have one or two cell types for which they are potent chemotactic factors. IL-8 is representative of this class in that it is primarily a chemotactic and activating factor for neutrophils in the pM-nM concentration range. IL-8 is also a chemotactic factor for T lymphocytes and stimulates endothelial cell proliferation.[26,27] At higher doses than those that are required for chemotaxis, IL-8 will stimulate neutrophils to degranulate and produce reactive oxygen metabolites.[28] IL-8 is also chemotactic for basophils and will stimulate the release of histamine.[29]

Monocyte chemoattractant protein-1 is similar to IL-8 in that it is produced by mononuclear phagocytes in response to similar stimuli.[30] However, the biologic activities of MCP-1 appear to be restricted to monocytes for which it is a chemotactic factor and will induce the respiratory burst. Recently, it has been shown that MCP-1 is sufficient for the induction of adhesion molecules expression as well as IL-1 and IL-6 production by monocytes.[31] Since IL-1 will in turn stimulate MCP-1 gene expression by the same cells, this may represent a potential positive feedback loop by which an initial pathologic stimulus may be amplified. MCP-1 also stimulates the cell surface expression of CD11b and CD11c, the alpha subunits of the integrin molecules MAC-1, and p150/95 on monocytes. These molecules form dimers with CD18 and mediate binding to stimulated endothelial cells.[32-34]

Anti-Inflammatory Cytokines

The third class of cytokines for which there is current evidence of involvement in HTRs may be considered as anti-inflammatory. Interleukin-1 receptor antagonist is a representative of this category. As with the other cytokines previously discussed, IL-1ra is produced by mononuclear phagocytes.[35] However, IL-1ra is quite different in that it appears to have no biologic activity in and of itself. Rather, IL-1ra is a competitive antagonist of IL-1 binding to type I cellular receptors.[36] IL-1ra will block the in-vivo and in-vitro effects of IL-1.[37] Thus, IL-1ra may prevent or down-regulate cellular activation events mediated by IL-1 in human disease states, including transfusion reactions.

Conclusions

To a large extent, the clinical variability of HTRs is likely explained by the relative balance of cytokine production in the transfusion recipient. Factors that increase the production of proinflammatory cytokines, such as complement fixation by alloantibodies or disease states such as sepsis, will tend to result in more severe reactions. The relative concentration of circulating chemokines that are produced as a primary response by phagocytes or derived from endothelium in response to proinflammatory cytokines will determine whether activated leukocytes will infiltrate target organs such as the kidney. Some HTRs, particularly those that result from IgG antibodies that do not fix complement, may be dominated by inhibitory cytokines such as IL-1ra that depress systemic responses. It such cases, relatively mild symptoms may be seen, despite clear evidence of immune hemolysis

References

1. Davenport RD. Hemolytic reactions. In: Popovsky MA, ed. Transfusion reactions. Bethesda, MD: AABB Press, 1996:25.
2. Davenport RD, Strieter RM, Kunkel SL. Red cell ABO incompatibility and production of tumour necrosis factor-alpha. Br J Haematol 1991; 78:540-4.
3. Butler J, Parker D, Pillai R, et al. Systemic release of neutrophil elastase and tumour necrosis factor alpha following ABO incompatible blood transfusion. Br J Haematol 1991;79:525-6.
4. Butler J, Parker D, Pillai R, et al. Effect of cardiopulmonary bypass on systemic release of neutrophil elastase and tumor necrosis factor. J Thorac Cardiovasc Surg 1993;105:25-30.
5. Davenport RD, Burdick M, Moore SA, Kunkel SL. Cytokine production in IgG-mediated red cell incompatibility. Transfusion 1993; 33:19-24.
6. Hoffman M. Antibody-coated erythrocytes induce secretion of tumor necrosis factor by human monocytes: A mechanism for the production of fever by incompatible transfusions. Vox Sang 1991;60:184-7.
7. Davenport RD, Strieter RM, Standiford TJ, Kunkel SL. Interleukin-8 production in red blood cell incompatibility. Blood 1990;76:2439-42.

8. Davenport RD, Burdick MD, Strieter RM, Kunkel SL. Monocyte chemoattractant protein production in red cell incompatibility. Transfusion 1994;34:16-9.
9. Ruegg SJ, Jungi TW. Antibody-mediated erythrolysis and erythrophagocytosis by human monocytes, macrophages and activated macrophages. Evidence for distinction between involvement of high-affinity and low-affinity receptors for IgG by using different erythroid target cells. Immunology 1988;63:513-20.
10. Leslie RGQ. Immunoglobulin and soluble immune complex binding to phagocyte Fc receptors. Biochem Soc Trans 1994;12:743-6.
11. Unkeless JC. Function and heterogeneity of human Fc receptors for immunoglobulin G. J Clin Invest 1989;83:355-61.
12. Clarkson SB, Kimberly RP, Valinsky JE, et al. Blockade of clearance of immune complexes by anti-Fc gamma receptor monoclonal antibody. J Exp Med 1986;164:474-89.
13. Clarkson SB, Bussel JB, Kimberly RP, et al. Treatment of refractory immune thrombocytopenic purpura with an anti-Fc gamma-receptor antibody. N Engl J Med 1986;314:1236-9.
14. Davenport RD, Kunkel SL. IgG receptor roles in red cell binding to monocytes and macrophages (abstract). Transfusion 1994;34 (suppl): 79S.
15. Davenport RD, Burdick MD, Strieter RM, Kunkel SL. In vitro production of Interleukin-1 receptor antagonist in IgG mediated red cell incompatibility. Transfusion 1994;34:297-303.
16. Okusawa S, Gelfand JA, Ikejima T, et al. Interleukin 1 induces a shock-like state in rabbits. Synergism with tumor necrosis factor and the effect of cyclooxygenase inhibition. J Clin Invest 1988;81:1162-72.
17. Freedman AS, Freeman G, Whitman J, et al. Pre-exposure of human B cells to recombinant IL-1 enhances subsequent proliferation. J Immunol 1988;141:3398-404.
18. Jelinek DF, Lipsky PE. Enhancement of human B cell proliferation and differentiation by tumor necrosis factor-alpha and interleukin 1. J Immunol 1987;139:2970-6.
19. Hackett RJ, Davis LS, Lipsky PE. Comparative effect of tumor necrosis factor-alpha and IL-1 beta on mitogen-induced T cell activation. J Immunol 1988;140:2639-44.
20. Muraguchi A, Hirano T, Tang B, et al. The essential role of B cell stimulatory factor 2 (BSF-2/IL-6) for the terminal differentiation of B cells. J Exp Med 1988;167:332-44.

21. Takatsuki F, Okano A, Suzuki C, et al. Human recombinant IL-6/B cell stimulatory factor 2 augments murine antigen-specific antibody responses in vitro and in vivo. J Immunol 1988;141:3072-7.
22. Matsuda T, Hirano T, Kishimoto T. Establishment of an interleukin 6 (IL-6)/B cell stimulatory factor 2-dependent cell line and preparation of anti-IL-6 monoclonal antibodies. Eur J Immunol 1988; 18:951-6.
23. Baroja ML, Ceuppens JL, Van Damme J, Billiau A. Cooperation between an anti-T cell (anti-CD28) monoclonal antibody and monocyte-produced IL-6 in the induction of T cell responsiveness to IL-2. J Immunol 1988;141:1502-7.
24. Garman RD, Jacobs KA, Clark SC, Raulet DH. B-cell-stimulatory factor 2 (beta$_2$ interferon) functions as a second signal for interleukin 2 production by mature murine T cells. Proc Natl Acad Sci USA 1987;84: 7621-33.
25. Helle M, Boeije L, Aarden LA. IL-6 is an intermediate in IL-1-induced thymocyte proliferation. J Immunol 1989;142:4335-8.
26. Houssiau FA, Coulie PG, Olive D, Van Snick J. Synergistic activation of human T cells by interleukin 1 and interleukin 6. Eur J Immunol 1988;18:653-8.
27. Larsen CG, Anderson AO, Appella E, et al. The neutrophil activating protein (NAP-1) is also chemotactic for T lymphocytes. Science 1989;243:1464-6.
28. Koch AE, Polverini PJ, Kunkel SL, et al. Interleukin-8 as a macrophage-derived mediator of angiogenesis. Science 1992;258:1798-801.
29. Matsushima K, Oppenheim JJ. Interleukin 8 and MCAF: Novel inflammatory cytokines inducible by IL 1 and TNF. Cytokine 1989;1:2-13.
30. White MV, Yoshimura T, Hook W, et al. Neutrophil attractant protein-1 (NAP-1) causes human basophil histamine release. Immunol Lett 1989;22:151-4.
31. Matsushima K, Larsen CG, DuBois GC, Oppenheim JJ. Purification and characterization of a novel monocyte chemotactic and activating factor produced by a human myelomonocytic cell line. J Exp Med 1989;169:1485-90.
32. Jiang Y, Beller DI, Frendl G, Graves DT. Monocyte chemoattractant protein-1 regulates adhesion molecule expression and cytokine production in human monocytes. J Immunol 1992;148:2423-8.
33. Butcher EC. Leukocyte-endothelial cell recognition: Three (or more) steps to specificity and diversity. Cell 1991;67:1033-6.

34. Stacker SA, Springer TA. Leukocyte integrin P150,95 (CD11c/CD18) functions as an adhesion molecule binding to a counter-receptor on stimulated endothelium. J Immunol 1991;146:648-55.
35. Arend WP, Joslin FG, Thompson RC, Hannum CH. An IL-1 inhibitor from human monocytes. Production and characterization of biologic properties. J Immunol 1989;143:1851-8.
36. Hannum CH, Wilcox CJ, Arend WP, et al. Interleukin-1 receptor antagonist activity of a human interleukin-1 inhibitor. Nature 1990;343: 336-40.
37. Ohlsson K, Bjork P, Bergenfeldt M, et al. Interleukin-1 receptor antagonist reduces mortality from endotoxin shock. Nature 1990;348: 550-2.

In: Davenport RD, Snyder EL, eds.
Cytokines in Transfusion Medicine: A Primer
Bethesda, MD: AABB Press, 1997

5

Erythropoietin in Blood Transfusion

MARIAN PETRIDES, MD

ERYTHROPOIETIN (EPO) IS A 30,400-DALTON GLYCOprotein that fosters maturation of bone marrow erythroid progenitors in response to hypoxic stimuli. Over the last two decades, much has been learned about the structure, regulation, and function of EPO. With the cloning of the EPO gene, it became possible to develop recombinant human erythropoietin (rhEPO) for therapeutic use. Since rhEPO became available for the treatment of anemia, clinical data have been accumulating concerning its efficacy in a variety of anemic states. Following a brief review of the physiology of EPO, this chapter summarizes the current state of the art with respect to the clinical indications, efficacy, and side effects of rhEPO therapy.

Marian Petrides, MD, Assistant Professor of Pathology and Director, Blood Bank, University of Mississippi Medical Center, Jackson, Mississippi

Structure and Physiology of Erythropoietin

The EPO gene is located on chromosome 7 and consists of five exons that code for a 166-amino acid protein. EPO, the protein product of this gene, is heavily glycosylated in humans. This glycosylation stabilizes the tertiary structure of the protein and is required for proper functioning in humans. EPO is highly conserved in nature, but the level of glycosylation varies considerably, with full glycosylation being found only in mammals. As a result, a mammalian expression system is required for the production of functional rhEPO.[1] The carbohydrate moiety of glycosylated EPO is rich in sialic acid residues that function to prevent hepatic clearance. While glycosylation is critical to EPO function, the absence of terminal sialic acid residues per se affects neither the tertiary structure of the molecule nor its binding to the EPO receptor.[2] The hydrophobic nature of the rhEPO molecule necessitates its stabilization in albumin to prevent adherence to glass surfaces. Studies using antipeptide antibodies have demonstrated that the carboxy-terminal end of the EPO molecule is responsible for binding EPO to its receptor.[1]

There are no preformed stores of EPO; rather, EPO is produced in response to hypoxic stimuli. Plasma levels of EPO normally bear an inverse relationship to hemoglobin or hematocrit, and consistently rise outside the normal range only when hemoglobin falls below 10.5 g/dL.[3] Animal studies have shown that anemia, hypoxia, and increased hemoglobin affinity for oxygen result in increased transcription, ie, increased EPO RNA, with a resultant increase in EPO production. In severely hypoxic animals, EPO levels peak at 12 hours, declining thereafter to half maximal levels even in the face of continued hypoxia. Furthermore, studies in hepatic cell lines have delineated induction of a hypoxia-inducible factor 1 (HIF-1) in response to hypoxia, which then binds to an enhancer located in the 3′ flanking region of the EPO gene. Binding of HIF-1 to this hypoxia-inducible enhancer then results in the activation of EPO transcription. The EPO promoter, which establishes initiation and orientation of transcription, has binding sites for HIF-1 and may play a minor role, acting in synergy with the EPO enhancer, in the induction of EPO transcription.[4]

In adults, EPO is produced primarily in the peritubular interstitial cells of the kidney, but in the developing fetus, EPO production takes place in the liver until late in gestation when there is a gradual shift away from hepatic production and toward renal synthesis. Once formed, EPO is transported via the circulation to the marrow. Binding of EPO to its receptor is critical to its function, and those erythroid progenitors that are most responsive to EPO [colony-forming unit-erythroid (CFU-E) and proerythroblasts] have the highest expression of EPO receptors on their cell surface.

The exact mechanism by which the binding of EPO to its receptor results in proliferation and maturation of red cell progenitors remains uncertain. Some workers postulate that EPO stimulates the synthesis of red-cell-specific proteins, such as spectrin and the globins. Others maintain that EPO merely acts to inhibit apoptosis (programmed cell death), thereby indirectly allowing enough time for these proteins to be expressed.[5] In any event, it appears clear that EPO results in both the proliferation and survival of immature red cell precursors, resulting in an increase in mature red cells and, thus, an increased red cell mass.

As a pharmacologic preparation, rhEPO is dispensed in vials of 2000 U, 3000 U, 5000 U, and 10,000 U and, as noted above, is generally stabilized in albumin to prevent adherence to glass surfaces and/or plastic tubing as a result of the hydrophobic nature of the molecule.

rhEPO in Renal Disease

An estimated 25% of renal dialysis patients require red cell transfusions,[6] and severe anemia is one of the major impediments to rehabilitation of these patients despite effective dialysis.[6,7] The anemia of end-stage renal disease is hypoproliferative and is characterized by very low levels of endogenous EPO because of the inability of the diseased kidney to produce adequate EPO. While other factors such as iron deficiency, hypersplenism, aluminum-induced toxic effects on red cells, blood loss via dialysis or the gastrointestinal tract, and possibly even circulating inhibitors to EPO may play a role, the primary cause of anemia in uremic patients remains the low endogenous secretion of EPO.[8,9] As a consequence, one would anticipate that treatment with rhEPO would be highly effective in reversing anemia in this setting, and studies over the last 10 years have shown this to be the case.[6,7]

Laboratory Effects

During 1986 and 1987, preliminary (Phase I-II) clinical trials of rhEPO in 25 severely anemic dialysis patients demonstrated a uniform, dose-dependent response in hematocrit to doses above 15 U/kg given intravenously three times weekly.[6] Doses below this threshold did not result in consistent changes in reticulocyte count or hematocrit, but, of the 18 patients who received effective doses, all demonstrated both a rise in hematocrit and elimination of the need for transfusion. The rate of increase in hematocrit was greatest with the largest doses (up to 500 U/kg three times weekly); patients receiving high-dose EPO were able to increase their hematocrit by as much as 10% over a period of 3 weeks.

In a follow-up Phase III multicenter clinical trial, 333 hemodialysis patients with uncomplicated anemia were treated with one of three different dose regimens of rhEPO, each given three times a week intravenously during the acute phase, followed by a maintenance dose of 75 U/kg three times weekly.[7] rhEPO dosing was adjusted in increments of 12.5-25 U/kg to maintain a stable hematocrit of 32-38%. The acute response rate was in excess of 97%, and virtually all of these patients were able to maintain a hematocrit in the target range without transfusion. Thirty-five patients received 300 U/kg per dose throughout the acute phase, 201 patients were given 150 U/kg throughout the acute phase, and 97 patients were treated with 300 U/kg initially, which was subsequently reduced to 150 U/kg while still in the acute phase. Overall, 97.4 % responded, demonstrating either a rise in hematocrit to 35% or an increase of 6% in hematocrit during the acute phase. Patients who received 150 U/kg during the acute phase showed about half the rate of increase in hematocrit seen in those treated with 300 U/kg while still in the acute phase. Those patients who did not respond were found to have additional causes beyond renal failure for anemia, including myelofibrosis or concomitant blood loss.

During the maintenance phase, the median dose required to maintain the hematocrit within the target range of 32-38% was 75 U/kg. Interestingly, while 83% of the patients could be maintained on 150 U/kg per dose or less, 17% required more than 150 U/kg to maintain a stable hematocrit for reasons that were not readily apparent. Patients' hemoglobin, hematocrit, and reticulocyte counts were monitored at 6 and 10 months following the start of maintenance therapy. By the end of the second month of the study, virtually all patients were transfusion-independent and remained so during the follow-up period. The only exceptions were in cases where there was either an interruption in the administration of rhEPO or blood loss during surgery or dialysis.

There was no evidence of either EPO resistance or the formation of antibodies directed against EPO. No significant change in white count was noted and, while the mean platelet count increased slightly but significantly during the acute phase, platelet counts still remained within the normal range and no further increase was noted during the maintenance phase.

In addition to being monitored with laboratory parameters such as hematocrit and reticulocyte counts, patients in this study were evaluated through the use of quality-of-life questionnaires. Most patients reported improved quality of life, with increased exercise tolerance, energy levels, and appetite.

Clinical Effects

Thirty-five percent of the patients in this study developed hypertension, which required an adjustment or institution of antihypertensive therapy in some cases.[7] The development of hypertension appeared to be unrelated to blood pressure at entry into the study. Several reasons have been proposed to explain the development of hypertension, including changes in blood viscosity and increased peripheral vascular resistance as a result of the reversal of the compensatory vasodilatation seen in anemia.[7,10,11] In any event, the development or exacerbation of hypertension does not appear to be a direct effect of rhEPO itself, since it has not been observed in populations without renal disease who are treated with rhEPO.[10]

Seizures occurred in 5.4% of patients. In some cases, seizures were related to the onset of uncontrolled hypertension (hypertensive encephalopathy). The incidence of seizures was comparable to that noted by others in dialysis patients not receiving rhEPO. Other adverse effects included absolute or functional iron deficiency in 43% of patients. The authors note that this figure would have been greater had not a fifth of the patients in the study been iron overloaded. Clotting of vascular access occurred in 39 patients (11.7%) who had a total of 60 thrombotic events, but this figure is comparable to that reported elsewhere in hemodialysis patients not receiving rhEPO. Myalgias and a flu-like syndrome temporally related to rhEPO administration were reported in 15 patients (4.5%).[7]

Subcutaneous vs Intravenous Administration of rhEPO

Most of the early work on EPO in renal disease utilized intravenous dosing regimens in hemodialysis patients, but studies involving peritoneal dialysis patients demonstrated that a subcutaneous route was feasible in this group,[12] whose hematocrits tend to be higher and who appear to have different EPO clearance kinetics. With subcutaneous administration, a much lower peak is achieved (20% of that obtained via the intravenous route) and peak levels are not reached until 12-24 hours. However, slow, continuous absorption from the subcutaneous injection site results in maintenance of EPO levels for up to 72 hours, compared with a half-life of 5-8 hours for EPO administered intravenously.[8] A randomized crossover study involving hemodialysis patients also concluded that subcutaneous and intravenous rhEPO are comparable both in effectiveness and in safety.[13]

The Effect of rhEPO in Predialysis and Dialysis Patients

Partly on the basis of results from animal studies as well as theoretical considerations, there was some concern that the use of rhEPO in predialysis renal patients might accelerate the progression of their disease to dialysis-dependence. Furthermore, it was known from earlier studies that dialyzable inhibitors of erythropoiesis are present in the serum of uremic patients, raising the question of whether rhEPO might be effective only in patients who were also being dialyzed and not in those who were not undergoing concomitant dialysis.[9]

Early randomized, placebo-controlled studies involving small numbers of predialysis patients with chronic renal insufficiency showed rhEPO to be effective in relieving anemia[14,15] without accelerating the progression of renal failure over the 12-week study period.[15] A large, multicenter, placebo-controlled, randomized, double-blind study subsequently demonstrated correction of anemia in rhEPO-treated patients significantly more frequently than that seen in placebo-treated controls (correction rate of 46-87%, depending on dose, in rhEPO-treated patients compared with 3% in placebo-treated patients[11]). During the 8-month course of the study, there was no evidence of accelerated deterioration of renal function in the rhEPO-treated arm when compared with placebo-treated controls.

Since the approval of rhEPO by the Food and Drug Administration in 1989, it has proved efficacious in raising hematocrit and reducing the need for transfusion in patients with renal failure, although response rates have been lower than anticipated because of the results seen in the clinical trials. By the end of 1993, 90% or more of dialysis patients were receiving rhEPO, as were 57% of peritoneal dialysis patients.[16] Several recent studies have found that 40-60% of dialysis patients receiving rhEPO in doses equivalent to those used in the clinical trials still failed to reach a hematocrit of 30%.[17,18] In terms of reduction in transfusion rate, a 6-year retrospective audit of transfusions to chronic hemodialysis patients found that significantly fewer red cell units were transfused per patient in 1991 than in 1988, the year prior to FDA approval of rhEPO (5.3 units compared with 8.6 units; $p<0.02$).[19] In addition, the frequency of red cell transfusions per 100 dialysis events was significantly lower in 1991 than in 1988 (4.11 compared with 13.35; $p<0.01$). Interestingly, however, only 24% of patients achieved transfusion independence during the 6-year study period.

In a search for the reasons why rhEPO fell short of expectations both in terms of the percentage of patients responding with hematocrits above 30% and in the proportion of patients achieving transfusion independence, Ifudu et al[18] examined the relationship between the intensity of hemodialysis and the response to rhEPO. Studying 145 hemodialysis patients receiving rhEPO in mean doses of 59 ± 29 U/kg three times weekly, the authors found that inadequate dialysis, defined as less than 65% reduction in blood urea nitrogen, was associated with a poor response to rhEPO. Increasing the urea-reduction value by 11% doubled the odds that a patient would achieve a hematocrit above 30%. Further testing this hypothesis, the authors then increased the intensity of dialysis for 6 weeks in the 20 patients who had baseline urea-reduction values less than 65%. Increasing the urea-reduction value from a mean of 60.7% to a mean of 72.0% in this group resulted in 70% of patients reaching a hematocrit greater than 30% compared with only 40% responding with hematocrits over 30% at the initial dialysis intensity. Thus, a failure to respond to rhEPO in dialysis-dependent renal failure may well be due to inadequate dialysis in many cases and, although still speculative, this may be the result of inadequate removal of uremic inhibitors of erythropoiesis.[8,9,18]

Summary

In conclusion, rhEPO has proven effective in raising hematocrit and reducing transfusion needs in renal failure patients. This is beneficial not only in terms of minimizing infectious disease exposure but also in decreasing the potential for sensitization to HLA-related antigens, which might interfere with subsequent renal transplantation.[19] While rhEPO can be given intravenously following hemodialysis, the subcutaneous route has been demonstrated to be equally effective and is more convenient in many cases, especially in patients who are not undergoing hemodialysis. Failure to respond and/or loss of responsiveness in a patient who has previously responded to rhEPO should precipitate a search for other complicating causes for anemia, such as blood loss or the development of functional iron deficiency. Adequacy of dialysis may also be a factor and should be considered when dialysis-dependent patients fail to respond to rhEPO.

rhEPO in the Anemia of Chronic Disease

The anemia of chronic disease (ACD) is a microcytic anemia characterized by diminished circulating iron (low serum iron and normal to decreased transferrin)[20] in the presence of adequate to increased iron stores. The name "anemia of chronic disease" is something of a misnomer because it is seen in a number of disease states most, but not all, of which are chronic. ACD is seen in chronic inflammatory states, such as rheumatoid arthritis, and in a variety of infections. It has been estimated to account for over half of the cases of anemia in which bleeding, hemolysis, and underlying hematologic malignancy have been ruled out, and some authorities feel that it may be second only to iron deficiency in frequency as a cause of anemia.[21]

The Pathogenesis of ACD

The pathogenesis of ACD is now well understood and is particularly instructive because many disease states that are associated with anemia, most notably cancer and human immunodeficiency virus (HIV) infection, are accompanied by some degree of chronic inflammation and may also present with intercurrent infection. Decreased red cell survival and impaired mobilization of iron from the reticuloendothelial system play a role in the pathogenesis of ACD, as do impaired production of and response to EPO. All of these are felt to be related to the presence of inflammatory cytokines.[21] In particular, cytokines appear to be responsible for both the submaximal production of EPO in response to anemia and the impaired response of erythroid progenitors to the EPO that is produced.

Impaired production of EPO has been documented in anemic cancer patients[22] and in patients with anemia resulting from rheumatoid arthritis.[23] Interleukin-1 (IL-1), tumor necrosis factor-α (TNF-α), and transforming growth factor-β (TGF-β) have been demonstrated to inhibit production of EPO in Hep 3B and Hep G2 cell lines and in isolated perfused rat kidneys. This effect appears to be at the level of mRNA.[24] However, even though EPO production in patients with ACD is less than it would be in simple iron deficiency anemia of the same severity, EPO levels are nonetheless higher than those in healthy, nonanemic individuals. There must, therefore, be some other mechanism at work as well.

Cytokines, namely, TNF, IL-1, and the interferons (IFNs), have all been shown to inhibit erythroid progenitor response to EPO. TNF inhibits CFU-E colony formation, apparently indirectly by a soluble factor released by marrow accessory cells in response to TNF. β-IFN, as well as another factor or factors, appear necessary for this inhibitory effect of TNF, as evidenced by the fact that neutralizing antibody to β-IFN eliminates the inhibitory effect of TNF. Further evidence of synergy comes from the observation that, while β-IFN has a direct effect on CFU-E colony formation, the amount of detectable β-IFN is insufficient to account for the degree of inhibition seen. The effect of IL-1 is likewise mediated by a soluble factor, in this case shown to be released by T lymphocytes, and the inhibition caused by IL-1 can be neutralized by antibody to γ-IFN. In vitro, this γ-IFN-mediated inhibition can be reversed by high doses of EPO. Finally, in vitro, these three classes of cytokines appear to act synergistically in inhibiting erythropoiesis.[24]

The role of cytokines in mediating impaired mobilization of iron in ACD is evidenced by the observation that rodents injected with recombinant TNF showed impaired release of iron from their reticuloendothelial system. Furthermore, IL-1 has been demonstrated to increase translation of ferretin mRNA, which has been postulated to act as a trap for iron that might otherwise be available for erythropoiesis.[24]

The Effectiveness of rhEPO Treatment

While most patients with ACD are only moderately anemic and may not benefit from rhEPO therapy, approximately 20-30% of ACD patients are sufficiently anemic to require red cell transfusion, and these patients may profit from treatment with rhEPO.[25] The first reported use of rhEPO in the setting of ACD was in 1989—two patients with rheumatoid arthritis received 100 U/kg three times weekly initially, followed by 150 U/kg. Both of these patients demonstrated correction of anemia with rhEPO therapy and recurrence of anemia on cessation of rhEPO.[26] A multicenter study[27] involving 17 rheumatoid arthritis patients confirmed this observation. Initially, four of 13 patients (30.7%) receiving intravenous rhEPO in doses of 50, 100, or 150 U/kg three times weekly showed a significant (6%) rise in hematocrit while none of the placebo-treated patients showed a significant hematocrit response. Eleven patients were then entered into an open label trial with rhEPO involving dose adjustment to allow maintenance of a hematocrit of 35% in women and 40% in men. Ten of the 11 (90.9%) attained the target hematocrit.

In addition, rhEPO may also have a place in the treatment of patients who require autologous blood donation and who would otherwise be unable to donate because of ACD. Thompson et al[28] reported a case of a 66-year-old man with a history of gastrointestinal bleeding as a result of esophageal varices who had previously developed multiple red cell alloantibodies and who, consequently, had a history of delayed hemolytic transfusion reactions. Administration of rhEPO allowed this patient to donate seven units of autologous blood before surgery for replacement of a prosthetic hip that was causing intractable pain. He required six of the seven units at surgery.

Finally, it is significant to note that rhEPO therapy for ACD has not been associated with increased incidence or exacerbations of hypertension or with hypertensive encephalopathy as it has been in patients with renal failure.[27,29] Dosages used in ACD are in the range of 50-150 U/kg three to five times weekly.

rhEPO in HIV Infection

Anemia is a common complication of HIV infection seen in three quarters of acquired immunodeficiency syndrome (AIDS) patients not receiving zidovudine (AZT).[30] Both the incidence and severity of anemia parallel the progression of the disease process.[30,31] Chronic inflammation, with elaboration of inflammatory cytokines that inhibit both EPO production and marrow responsiveness to EPO, and intercurrent infections play a role in the development of anemia in patients with HIV infection. As expected, therefore, serum levels of endogenous EPO have been demonstrated to be inappropriately low in the anemia in patients with untreated HIV infection, when compared with iron deficiency anemia of comparable severity.[30]

Treatment with AZT increases both the incidence and severity of anemia in AIDS patients.[32,33] In one study, severe anemia with hemoglobin levels below 7.5 g/dL was seen in 24% of AZT-treated AIDS patients and in only 4% of similar patients receiving a placebo ($p < 0.001$).[33] Over two-thirds of AZT-treated AIDS patients had endogenous EPO levels less than 500 IU/kg.[32]

The Effectiveness of rhEPO Treatment

The use of rhEPO has been studied both in HIV patients being treated with AZT and in patients infected with the virus but not receiving such treatment. In both groups of patients, rhEPO was shown to result in significant increases in hematocrit and significant reduction in transfusion rate, provided the patient's baseline endogenous EPO level was 500 IU/L or lower. Patients with endogenous EPO levels greater than 500 IU/L showed no benefit from rhEPO therapy.[32,34] Both clinical and in vitro studies have demonstrated no potentiation of HIV infection by rhEPO therapy.[32,34,35]

In an early randomized, double-blind, placebo-controlled trial,[36] the efficacy of 100 U/kg rhEPO given intravenously three times weekly was evaluated in 63 AIDS patients who were being treated with AZT. This study demonstrated a significant reduction in both transfusion rate (percent of patients requiring transfusion) and number of units transfused per month in patients whose baseline EPO levels were 500 IU/L or lower.

Henry et al[32] analyzed four, 12-week, randomized, double-blind, placebo-controlled studies involving a total of 297 AIDS patients receiving AZT therapy and reached similar conclusions. The four studies were similar in design and could therefore be combined and analyzed together. Patients were randomly selected to receive either a placebo or rhEPO, given intravenously or subcutaneously, in doses of 100-200 U/kg three times weekly. A little over two-thirds (69%) of the patients studied had baseline endogenous EPO levels 500 IU/L or lower. In these patients, rhEPO therapy resulted in a decrease in transfusion requirements by an average of two units over 3 months and an increase in hematocrit by an average of 4% when compared with placebo. Both the reduction in transfusion requirements (3.2 units for the rhEPO group compared with 5.3 units for the placebo; $p = 0.003$) and the increase in hematocrit (4.6% compared with 0.5%; $p<0.001$) were statistically significant. rhEPO was of no benefit to patients with baseline EPO levels greater than 500 IU/L.

No difference in adverse effects was found between rhEPO-treated patients and those treated with placebo. rhEPO did not result in significant change in blood pressure or in potentiation of HIV infection, as indicated by serum p24 antigen levels, total lymphocyte counts, or in vitro assays of HIV proliferation in infected cell lines.

A large multicenter open-label treatment protocol[34] conducted in 1943 anemic (hematocrit 30% or less) AIDS patients with endogenous EPO levels of 500 IU/L or lower confirmed that rhEPO was effective in increasing hematocrit and decreasing transfusion requirements, whether or not the patients were also receiving AZT. In this trial, subcutaneous rhEPO was given at a dose of 24,000 units weekly in six daily doses for an initial treatment period of 6-12 weeks. If the hematocrit failed either to rise by 6% or to reach the target range of 38-40%, the rhEPO dose was increased at 6-12-week intervals to a maximum of 48,000 units weekly. Mean hematocrit rose from a baseline of 28% to 33.1% at 12 weeks and 33.8% at week 24, and this increase was sustained throughout the study to week 54. During the 6-week period before the study, 40% of patients required at least one transfusion. At weeks 12 and 24, the percentage requiring transfusion fell to 22% and 18%, respectively. Forty-four percent of patients responded with both a rise in hematocrit of 6% or more over baseline and no need for transfusions within the 28-day period before reaching that hematocrit. Data from this protocol also confirm that effective doses range from 343-492 U/kg per week, which is consistent with recommended dosing guidelines of 100 U/kg three times weekly for an initial dose, with dose escalation to 300 U/kg three times weekly depending on response. Again, there was no evidence of an adverse effect of rhEPO therapy on disease progression, but hypertension was seen in 1% of patients and seizures were reported in 1%.

In addition to these clinical studies that showed no potentiation of HIV infection in the presence of rhEPO, in vitro studies in cultures of monocytes/macrophages have demonstrated that rhEPO has no effect on HIV replication. Similarly, in-vitro studies have found no adverse impact of rhEPO on the antiviral activity of the dideoxynucleosides used to treat HIV infection, AZT, 2´,3´- dideoxyinosine (ddI), and 2´,3´-dideoxycytidine (ddC).[35]

Combination Therapy With G-CSF and rhEPO

Treatment with AZT results in neutropenia as well as anemia and the neutropenia is potentially a greater threat to life than is the anemia. Theoretical concerns had been raised about the possibility that rhEPO might result in "lineage steal"[37] and reduce the effectiveness of concomitantly administered granulocyte colony-stimulating factor (G-CSF). Fortunately, however, this does not appear to be the case. In a trial by Miles et al,[38] 22 advanced-stage AIDS patients with leukopenia and anemia were treated with G-CSF followed by G-CSF plus rhEPO in doses up to 500 U/kg daily. All myelosuppressive medications had been discontinued at least 4 weeks before study entry. Normalization of neutrophil counts was seen in all patients within 48 hours of the start of G-CSF therapy. The addition of rhEPO resulted in both correction of anemia in all 20 evaluable patients and maintenance of normal neutrophil counts, demonstrating that combination therapy with G-CSF and rhEPO can be beneficial in treating both anemia and neutropenia in AIDS patients in the absence of AZT. Reintroduction of AZT resulted in anemia severe enough to require transfusion in eight of the 20 patients, despite continued G-CSF and rhEPO. Thus, 60% of the patients maintained on both G-CSF and rhEPO remained transfusion-independent following the reinstitution of AZT. No adverse effects on HIV replication were seen.

Summary

In summary, rhEPO in doses of 100-300 U/kg three times weekly is effective in both raising hematocrit and reducing transfusion requirements in HIV-infected patients whose endogeneous EPO levels are 500 U/L or less, whether or not these patients are being treated with AZT. In addition to reducing the potential for infectious disease exposure and diminishing the likelihood of transfusion reactions, decreasing transfusion rates in AIDS patients may also be beneficial in avoiding the down-regulation of the immune system that may accompany transfusion of allogeneic blood.[32] No evidence was found, either clinically or in in vitro studies, that rhEPO potentiates the replication of the HIV virus, nor does it interfere with concomitant administration of G-CSF for neutropenia. Hypertension and seizures were seen in a small number (1%) of patients, although the latter may have been due to the underlying HIV infection in at least some cases.

rhEPO in Cancer and Myelodysplastic Syndromes

The anemia seen in cancer patients is multifactorial in origin, with ACD, chemotherapy, and radiation effects on marrow, marrow invasion by tumor, and subclinical hemolysis[39,40] all potentially playing a role. Current evidence suggests that a blunted endogenous EPO response may well mediate a number of these causes for anemia. Miller et al[22] studied 81 adult patients with solid tumors and anemia and found that these patients had inappropriately low serum endogenous EPO levels for any given degree of anemia when compared with 24 control patients with similar levels of anemia resulting from iron deficiency. The blunting of EPO production in response to anemia was further exacerbated in patients who were undergoing concomitant chemotherapy. In addition, they noted that anemic cancer patients lose the inverse correlation usually seen between hemoglobin concentration and endogenous EPO levels. On the other hand, anemic cancer patients still appear to be capable of responding to hypoxic challenge with adequate production of endogenous EPO. Cancer patients who were both hypoxic and anemic demonstrated EPO levels similar to those seen in iron-deficient controls and, as expected, showed an inverse correlation between hemoglobin level and EPO concentration.

rhEPO in Patients With Solid Tumors

In view of this relative deficiency of endogenous EPO, it seemed likely that anemic cancer patients might respond to treatment with rhEPO and, indeed, early dose-escalation trials reported response rates ranging from 50-85%.[41,42] A series of three, randomized, double-blind, placebo-controlled trials were conducted on a total of 413 patients to elucidate further the response of anemia to rhEPO therapy in cancer patients.[43] In the first of these studies, patients who had received no chemotherapy (No CTX) were given either 100 U/kg of rhEPO or a placebo subcutaneously three times a week for up to 8 weeks. The other two trials were conducted on patients receiving chemotherapy, with cisplatin (CTX-PLAT) or without cisplatin (CTX only). Presumably, the rationale for studying cisplatin-containing regimens separately from the larger chemotherapy group lies in the observation of a decrease in EPO response to anemia in patients receiving cisplatin,[22] which is nephrotoxic. In both of the chemotherapy trials, a higher dose and longer duration of rhEPO were used, namely, 150 U/kg subcutaneously three times a week for 12 weeks.

In all three groups, the mean increase in hematocrit seen in the rhEPO-treated arm of the study was significantly greater ($p<0.04$) than that seen in the placebo arm (2.8% compared with –0.1% in the No-CTX group, 6.9% compared with 1.1% in the CTX-only group and 6.0% compared with 1.3% in the CTX-PLAT group). Furthermore, when the two chemotherapy trials were combined and analyzed together, rhEPO-treated patients had significantly lower transfusion requirements after the first month than did control patients. In rhEPO-treated chemotherapy patients, 27.8% were transfused during the second and third months of the study compared with 45.5% of controls ($p<0.05$), and the mean number of units transfused was 1.04 in the rhEPO patients compared with 1.81 for control patients ($p = 0.009$). This effect did not extend to patients not receiving chemotherapy and did not reach the level of statistical significance if the two chemotherapy groups were analyzed separately. Finally, in a quality-of-life assessment, rhEPO-treated patients who demonstrated a 6% or greater rise in hematocrit indicated a significant improvement in energy level, ability to do activities of daily living, and overall quality of life when compared with those who received placebo ($p<0.05$).

Although there was no statistically significant difference in the incidence of any adverse effect in the rhEPO arm, hypertension was noted to occur "occasionally" in rhEPO-treated patients, generally in association with rises in hematocrit to levels significantly above normal. In a separate report on the CTX-only study,[29] while there was no statistically significant difference in the incidence of hypertension as an adverse effect (4/81 rhEPO-treated patients compared with 2/76 controls), the hypertension seen in rhEPO-treated patients was noted to be more severe than in placebo-treated patients. In this same report, equal numbers of patients (two in each study arm) had seizures during therapy. Seizures in the rhEPO-treated patients occurred in the context of significant rises in both hematocrit and blood pressure, but these same patients also had structural abnormalities of the central nervous system.

Following completion of the double-blind phase of the above studies, 363 patients were entered into an open-label follow-up study[43] in which the dose was adjusted to a maximum of 900 U/kg per week to achieve and maintain a target hematocrit of 38%. Response was defined as an increase of at least 6% in hematocrit without transfusion in the preceding month, and a complete response was defined as achievement of the target hematocrit without transfusion in the preceding month. During the entire course of rhEPO therapy, response rates were 40.0%, 56.1%, and 58.3% in the No-CTX, CTX-only, and CTX-PLAT groups, respectively, with average weekly doses of 382 U/kg, 513 U/kg, and 488 U/kg, respectively. In patients who received rhEPO for more than 12 weeks, response rates were higher: 57.9% (No-CTX), 63.5% (CTX only), and 70.2% (CTX-PLAT). The percentage of patients transfused fell over 6 months of therapy from 31.4% to 10.3% in the No-CTX group, 25.2% to 13.0% in the CTX-only group, and 42.7% to 11.5% in the CTX-PLAT group.

Thus, the largest multicenter trial to date demonstrated that rhEPO, generally in doses under 500 U/kg per week, resulted in significant increases in hematocrit in anemic cancer patients. Response rates ranged from 40-70% depending on the nature of concomitant chemotherapy, if any, and on the duration of rhEPO therapy. Higher response rates were seen in patients receiving concomitant chemotherapy, especially with cisplatin-containing regimens. Decreases in transfusion requirements were also noted, although the latter effect required a lag of about 1 month before it was demonstrable.

It is apparent from the above trials that a significant proportion (30-60%) of anemic cancer patients will not respond to rhEPO. Therefore, it would be advantageous, both to the patient and from a cost-containment standpoint, to be able to predict which anemic cancer patients are likely to respond to rhEPO. In the preceding study, patients not receiving chemotherapy who had baseline endogenous EPO below 100 U/L or ferretin levels less than 400-500 ng/mL appeared to have somewhat higher response rates. Neither pretreatment endogenous EPO levels nor pretreatment ferretin levels were of predictive value in chemotherapy patients.

Early rise in hemoglobin or reticulocyte count appeared to be better predictors of response, particularly when both were present simultaneously. In patients receiving chemotherapy, those who demonstrated a rise in hemoglobin of at least 1 gm/dL or a 40,000/µL or greater increase in reticulocyte count at 4 weeks from inception of therapy had a response rate of 84%. Similarly, in patients not receiving chemotherapy, a 0.5 gm/dL or greater rise in hemoglobin or a 40,000/µL or greater increase in reticulocytes was accompanied by response in 91%.[44]

Ludwig et al[45] also looked for predictors of response in 80 patients treated with 150 U/kg subcutaneous rhEPO initially, with dose increases to 300 U/kg in those who failed to respond in 6 weeks. They likewise found baseline EPO, ferretin, iron, transferrrin, and transferrin receptors to be incapable of predicting response to rhEPO, but an early rise in hemoglobin or a fall in ferretin were predictive. Specifically, they found that in responders the serum EPO level remains stable while the hemoglobin rises by 0.5 gm/dL or more in the first two weeks of therapy, suggesting consumption of exogenous EPO. EPO accumulates rather than being consumed in nonresponders, resulting in an increase in serum EPO level without a significant rise in hemoglobin. Alternatively, they found that a serum ferretin of 400 ng/mL or more after 2 weeks of rhEPO therapy was a strong indicator of unresponsiveness.

Multiple myeloma and myelodysplastic syndromes (MDS) merit separate consideration, because there has naturally been some concern that treatment with rhEPO in the setting of hematologic malignancy and/or premalignant states might stimulate the progression of disease. Furthermore, patients with these two diagnoses have been found to respond to rhEPO differently from the general cancer population and from each other, with myeloma patients showing a dramatically greater response rate than other cancer patients[39,46] and myelodysplastic patients demonstrating very poor response rates.[47]

rhEPO in Patients With Multiple Myeloma

In a pilot study on the use of rhEPO in patients with multiple myeloma, Ludwig et al[39] treated 13 patients with rhEPO for 6 months with an intial dose of 150 U/kg subcutaneously three times weekly, with dose escalation in 50 U/kg increments to a maximum of 250 U/kg three times weekly in nonresponders. Eleven of the 13 (85%) responded with a 2 g/dL or greater rise in hemoglobin, most (nine patients) within the first 2 months of therapy. Pretreatment endogenous EPO levels were higher in late responders and in nonresponders than they were in patients with a timely response, all of whom had baseline endogenous EPO levels less than 100 U/L. Because, for the purposes of this study, any transfusion was deemed to represent a failure to respond, all responders were, by definition, transfusion-free during the course of the study. No adverse effects were noted in any patient.

Beyond providing data that patients with multiple myeloma show a very high response rate, even in the absence of renal failure (all but one of the patients studied had normal renal function), this study also provides evidence that rhEPO therapy does not result in proliferation of the malignant plasma-cell clone. Quantitative immunoglobulins were obtained during therapy with rhEPO and compared with pretreatment levels as a measure of the impact of rhEPO on serum M component. No obvious differences were noted, and there was no statistically significant trend in the serum M component during treatment with rhEPO. In addition, there was no significant difference in the extent of bone marrow infiltration by myeloma cells when pretreatment marrows were compared with marrows obtained following 3 months of rhEPO therapy.

A follow-up study[46] of similar design involving 28 patients with multiple myeloma revealed a similar response rate. Sixty percent of patients showed a brisk response within the first month of treatment with 150 U/kg of subcutaneous rhEPO three times weekly and, overall, 75% responded with a 2 g/dL or greater rise in hemoglobin. This study did not provide for dose escalation in nonresponders, which might well have resulted in an even higher overall response rate because an unspecified number of nonresponders showed a 1 g/dL rise in hemoglobin but failed to reach the 2 g/dL threshold used to define response. Again, high baseline endogenous EPO levels (greater than 100 U/L) predicted late response or no response. Another indicator of likelihood of response appeared to be the nature of the treatment that patients were receiving for their myeloma because patients on alkylating agents tended to show a less rapid response than those treated with autologous marrow transplants and with interferon.

rhEPO in Patients With Myelodysplastic Syndromes

In contrast with the dramatically high response rates seen in myeloma, rhEPO therapy alone resulted in response rates of less than 20% in patients with MDS. In 1993, Greenberg summarized data from seven studies and found that only 14/75 (19%) of patients responded to rhEPO in total weekly doses ranging from a 150-3,000 U/kg.[48] The highest response rate (42%) noted was in a study utilizing 200-1,000 U/kg intravenously three times weekly, with other studies using lower doses yielding responses in 7-25% of patients.[48] Data from an eighth study[49] has brought the total number treated to 84, 19 of whom responded, for an overall response rate of 23%.

The observation that EPO and G-CSF can have a synergistic effect on erythropoiesis in vitro led to a trial of sequential G-CSF followed by rhEPO plus G-CSF in 28 patients with MDS,[49] five of whom had previously failed to respond to rhEPO alone. In this study, 42% of patients responded to combination therapy with G-CSF and subcutaneous rhEPO given at an initial dose of 100 U/kg daily, with dose escalation to 300 U/kg daily. Responses appeared to be independent of FAB subclass, but baseline endogenous EPO levels were significantly lower in responders than in nonresponders. There was, however, substantial overlap between the range for endogenous EPO levels in responders and in nonresponders. Numerous questions remain unanswered at this time regarding the combined use of G-CSF and rhEPO in MDS patients, including the durabilty of response and, more importantly, the impact of such therapy on the progression of MDS.

By far the largest study to date was a recently reported, open-label, multicenter trial involving 116 patients with MDS in which rhEPO alone was used at an initial dose of 150 U/kg three times weekly, with dose escalations of 50 U/kg monthly in nonresponders to a maximum dose of 300 U/kg thrice weekly. Response was defined as either a 6% or greater increase in hematocrit without transfusion or a 50% decline in transfusion requirements. The overall response rate (28%) was comparable to that previously reported, but the interesting finding was that the group who were responders had a noticeably higher proportion of patients with FAB classification of refractory anemia (RA) than did the nonresponder group (60% compared with 38%; difference not statistically significant). Furthermore, the mean baseline EPO level was significantly lower in responders than in nonresponders (70.4 U/L compared with 168.1 U/L; $p < 0.05$). The overall response rate among patients with a diagnosis of refractory anemia was 38%, but 54% of patients with RA and a baseline endogenous EPO level of 100 U/L or lower responded to rhEPO.[50] Thus, whereas the overall response rate in patients with MDS remains low, the subset of patients who both carry the diagnosis of RA and who have low (≤100 U/L) baseline endogenous EPO levels appear to have a reasonable likelihood of responding to rhEPO in doses ranging from 150-300 U/kg three times a week.

rhEPO in Patients Undergoing Bone Marrow Transplantation

The use of rhEPO in bone marrow transplantation, yet another setting in which endogenous EPO levels have been found to be inappropriately low,[51-53] represents a final special case to consider. In the largest, randomized, double-blind, placebo-controlled multicenter clinical trial to date,[54] 91 patients receiving allogeneic marrow transplants from identical sibling donors were treated with either a placebo or rhEPO 300 U/kg three times weekly via the intravenous route. While rhEPO-treated patients had significantly higher hemoglobin levels and reticulocyte counts after 14 days of treatment ($p<0.0005$), multivariate analysis was required before a statistical difference in the number of red cell units transfused or in the transfusion rate could be appreciated. Controls required 7 ± 5 units of packed red cells compared with 6 ± 5 in the rhEPO-treated group. The transfusion rate for controls was 19% compared with 16% for patients being treated with rhEPO. When multivariate analysis was performed, these data revealed an 18% reduction in transfusion requirements in patients treated with rhEPO, although the authors felt that this was not clinically significant enough to be cost-effective. Similarly, a randomized, placebo-controlled trial[55] in allogeneic marrow recipients utilizing either a placebo or 200 U/kg intravenous rhEPO daily for 4 weeks followed by 200 U/kg twice weekly for an additional 4 weeks demonstrated significantly higher hemoglobin levels at 2 months ($p = 0.020$) and significantly lower transfusion requirements during the first 2 months (5 units compared with 10 units; $p = 0.04$) in rhEPO-treated patients.

Preliminary data in autologous marrow transplant recipients are not as encouraging, with several studies reporting no significant difference in transfusion requirements between placebo-treated controls and rhEPO-treated patients.[56-59] One possible reason for this disparity between autologous and allogeneic transplant patients may be that recipients of allogeneic marrow are more likely to demonstrate inappropriately low endogenous EPO response to anemia than are patients undergoing autologous rescue with either marrow or peripheral blood progenitor cells.[52,53]

rhEPO in the Anemia of Prematurity

An estimated 80% of very low-birth-weight infants (<1250 g) require transfusion[60] because of 1) iatrogenic blood loss as the result of phlebotomy and 2) the normal physiologic drop in hematocrit seen postnatally in all infants as a result of the rapid expansion of blood volume, which accompanies rapid growth in neonates. The physiologic anemia of infancy rarely results in a hemoglobin of less than 9 g/dL in healthy term neonates and, therefore, rarely presents a problem. In premature infants, however, mean hemoglobin levels drop considerably lower, as low as a mean of 7 g/dL in the population weighing less than 1 kg at birth.[61] This so-called "anemia of prematurity" is characterized by reticulocytopenia, marrow hypoplasia, and relatively low endogenous EPO levels for the degree of anemia. Current evidence suggests that low EPO production is the primary cause of the anemia of prematurity, not diminished response of erythroid progenitors to EPO.[61,62] Thus, one would anticipate that rhEPO would be effective in this setting.

The Effectiveness of rhEPO Treatment

Early trials failed to show a clear benefit to the use of rhEPO in very low-birth-weight infants,[63] perhaps because doses of rhEPO (200 U/kg weekly) were suboptimal. Subsequently, however, several randomized, controlled studies,[64-66] including two large multicenter clinical trials[62,67] have demonstrated a small but significant reduction in transfusion needs of rhEPO-treated neonates.

In a multicenter trial conducted at 11 US sites,[62] a total of 157 newborns with a birth weight of 1250 g or less and gestational age of less than 31 weeks were entered into the study at an average of 3 weeks of age. They were randomly selected to receive either a placebo or a weekly dose of 500 U/kg of rhEPO, given in five divided doses, for 6 weeks. In order to avoid confounding variables related to phlebotomy losses in unstable infants, only clinically stable infants with phlebotomy requirements of less than 7.5

mL per week were enrolled. In a departure from other studies, otherwise stable infants with ongoing medical problems, including those who required ventilator or continuous positive airway pressure support, were not excluded. All infants received oral iron supplements, equivalent to 3 mg/kg/day of elemental iron initially, with an increase to 6 mg/kg/day when tolerating full caloric feedings. Infants in both groups were transfused in accordance with a set of specific indications for transfusion that was established for the study.

During the study period of 6 weeks, newborns who were treated with rhEPO received significantly fewer red cell transfusions than did the infants supported by transfusion alone (mean = 1.1 per patient compared with 1.6 per patient; p = 0.046) and the volume of packed red cells transfused was smaller in the rhEPO group than in the placebo group (mean = 16.5 mL compared with 23.9 mL; p = 0.023). Reticulocyte count and hematocrit were likewise significantly higher in the rhEPO group (p = 0.0001 in both cases).

More rhEPO-treated infants avoided transfusion during the study period (43% compared with 31%); this was statistically significant only when subjected to multiple logistic regression. If transfusions received prior to entry into the study are included, patients in the rhEPO group received a mean of 4.4 red cell transfusions per patient, whereas the placebo group required a mean of 5.3 transfusions per patient. This amounts to a 31% reduction in transfusion requirements during the study period, a 17% reduction in transfusion requirements overall and, most important, approximately one less red cell transfusion per infant in the rhEPO-treated group.

A multicenter European trial[67] arrived at similar conclusions regarding the efficacy of rhEPO. In this study, 241 infants with a birth weight of 750-1499 g and a gestational age of 34 weeks or less were randomly selected to receive either 750 U/kg of rhEPO weekly in three divided doses along with oral iron supplements or iron alone. Initial iron doses were 2 mg per day beginning on day 14, with dose increases in the event of a fall in serum ferretin level and/or the development of signs of iron deficiency. Success, defined as the absence of transfusion requirement and a hematocrit that never fell below 32%, was achieved by 27.5% of the rhEPO-treated infants, compared with only 4.1% of the control infants. Likewise, the mean number of red cell transfusions was significantly lower in the rhEPO group than in the control group (0.87 transfusion per patient compared with 1.25 transfusions per patient; p = 0.013).

Clinical Utility and Cost-Effectiveness

Despite the observation in these two large multicenter trials that rhEPO does, in fact, result in significant reduction in red cell transfusions in very low-birth-weight infants, numerous questions remain concerning the clinical utility and cost-effectiveness of rhEPO in the anemia of prematurity. While a number of authors have concluded that rhEPO is both efficacious[62,65-68] and cost-effective,[66,67] others disagree. In particular, Fain et al[60] applied decision analysis and sensitivity analysis to the data from the US multicenter study and found that rhEPO used in conjunction with transfusion was considerably more expensive than transfusion alone (3.6 times as costly over the 6-week study period). They concluded that rhEPO as used in the US multicenter study was not cost-effective for widespread use in treating the anemia of prematurity.

A significant problem with the costs for rhEPO in the US study was the enormous waste of rhEPO that occurred because each dose was taken from a separate 2000 U vial and the average dose administered was 140 U. Using each vial for multiple doses was not possible because the product contains no preservative and, thus, the manufacturer's instructions specifically state that the vial is to be entered only once and the contents, once withdrawn, must be used within 24 hours. A significant reduction in cost could be effected if multidose vials with a longer shelf life were available. These studies also did not address the issue of whether using rhEPO in the first days of life might reduce the early transfusion rate and, therefore, result in a greater reduction in red cell transfusion and an improvement in cost-effectiveness.

One further consideration is whether altering current neonatal transfusion practices to allow the use of a single dedicated red blood cell unit until its expiration date might be as effective as, or more so than, rhEPO therapy. Transfusion to replace phlebotomy losses in very low-birth-weight infants often takes place in the first week or two of life,[69] before rhEPO can effect a rise in hematocrit.[70] In six separate studies cited by Hume and Bard,[69] the volume transfused could easily have been provided from a single unit from which aliquots were removed using a sterile connecting device. The use of a single packed red cell unit for the full 35 days of its shelf life has been demonstrated to be both safe and effective in meeting the needs of premature neonates.[71] Thus, if the red cell unit from which the original aliquot was taken were dedicated to that infant and used for further transfusions until its expiration, this would effectively limit the number of donor exposures in most cases to the single donor to whom the infant would have been exposed whether or not he/she had received rhEPO. This, of course, presumes that neonatologists, who have long been concerned about high potassium and low 2,3-diphosphoglycerate (2,3-DPG) levels in stored units, would be persuaded by the Liu study cited above to continue to use such a dedicated unit until its expiration.

rhEPO Side Effects Unique to Neonates

In any discussion of the use of rhEPO in neonates, one must also discuss the unique side effects seen when rhEPO is used in this population. Neutropenia has been reported in association with rhEPO therapy,[66] but this has not been reported to increase the risk of infection.[61] Interestingly, neutropenia was not observed in either of the large multicenter studies. There have also been several reports of sudden infant death syndrome (SIDS)[64,67,72] occurring weeks to months after hospital discharge, although these events could not be directly attributed to rhEPO. There were no cases of SIDS reported in the US multicenter study[62] and the three cases that occurred in the European multicenter study[67] were equally distributed between the rhEPO group (one case), the control group (one case), and the group of infants withdrawn from the study because of prolonged ventilator support (one case). Other risks mentioned include possible diminution of growth, increased levels of fetal hemoglobin (with resultant increase in oxygen affinity and decrease in oxygen delivery to the tissues), and a drug interaction with theophylline, which results in higher levels of rhEPO in neonates who receive the two drugs concomitantly.

In a study designed to assess the long-term impact as well as the short-term effects of rhEPO, Soubasi et al[65] randomly selected 97 infants into three groups: one group received rhEPO (750 U/kg per week) (EPO 750), and the second group received rhEPO (300 U/kg per week) (EPO 300), and the third group received no rhEPO (control). Infants in each group were treated for 6 weeks from the first week of life and then followed until 12 months of age. The mean number of red cell transfusions required from the discontinuation of rhEPO until discharge was significantly lower for both rhEPO groups when compared with untreated controls (0.38 and 0.52 for EPO 300 and EPO 750 compared with 0.9 for controls, $p<0.05$). Levels of hemoglobin F were significantly higher in both rhEPO groups at the end of treatment and until the third month of life, but at 3, 6, and 12 months of age, there were no significant differences in hemoglobin F, growth, or reticulocyte percentage among the three groups. Furthermore, rhEPO therapy did not suppress endogenous production of EPO following the discontinuation of rhEPO therapy.

Summary

In conclusion, it is clear that rhEPO does significantly reduce transfusion in very low-birth-weight infants, but the magnitude of that reduction remains small in most cases. As a consequence, rhEPO is not yet regarded as a standard treatment in the anemia of prematurity, especially since the risks of rhEPO in premature infants are not yet completely defined.[73] Furthermore, whether the use of rhEPO is cost-effective and whether the same therapeutic effect can be achieved by other methods remains to be seen. Future directions for study will likely include evaluation of the efficacy of rhEPO therapy if instituted earlier, ie, in the first several days of life, and consideration of the effect of restricting the use of rhEPO to that group of infants who are most likely to require transfusion.

rhEPO in the Perioperative Period

As concern about transfusion-associated infectious disease transmission has risen over the last decade, so has interest in alternatives to allogeneic blood transfusion for surgical patients. rhEPO has two potential roles in this setting: first, improving the yield of preoperative autologous blood donation (PAD) and, second, accelerating the recovery of hemoglobin postoperatively, thus reducing the need for transfusion.

Autologous blood donation has grown in popularity over the last decade to the point where it is now regarded as the standard of care in some elective surgical procedures.[74,75] However, 5-30% of patients who donate autologous blood preoperatively will also require allogeneic transfusion in the perioperative period.[74,76] The likelihood of this occurring obviously depends on the nature of the procedure and the blood loss associated with it, but the age, health, and predonation hematocrit of the patient undergoing the procedure are also factors.

Goodnough et al[77] looked at the impact of PAD on allogeneic blood exposure in 263 patients undergoing elective orthopedic surgery and found that allogeneic blood transfusion was more likely to occur in patients who either were requested to collect four or more units of autologous blood or who were anemic at the first donation. Seventeen percent (20/116) of the patients whose surgeons requested four or more autologous units required allogeneic transfusion as compared with only 2% (3/146) of those for whom three or fewer units were requested. Of the 67 patients who were anemic at their first donation, only 42% (28/67) successfully donated the number of units requested compared with 151 of the 196 patients (77%) who were not anemic. Furthermore, 27% of the patients with baseline anemia required allogeneic transfusion at surgery, compared with only 11% of those who were not anemic at first donation.

The Effect on Red Cell Collection and the Need for Allogeneic Transfusion

Autologous blood donors have been shown to exhibit insufficient endogenous EPO response to phlebotomy,[78,79] suggesting that they might benefit from rhEPO to enhance red cell collection. Several studies have shown that rhEPO can increase the volume of autologous blood that can be collected preoperatively[70,80-82] and also can reduce the risk of allogeneic blood exposure.[83] In a randomized, double-blind, placebo-controlled study[80] of 47 adults scheduled for elective orthopedic surgery, Goodnough et al found that rhEPO significantly improved the volume of blood that could be collected from patients undergoing aggressive (twice weekly for 3 weeks) phlebotomy for PAD.[80] All patients received oral iron supplements three times daily and patients in the rhEPO arm also received 600 U/kg of intravenous rhEPO at each visit, whether or not blood was actually collected. Patients were deferred from donation if they presented with a hematocrit less than 34%. The mean red cell volume donated by patients receiving rhEPO therapy was 41% higher than that donated by patients receiving only iron (961 mL compared with 683 mL, $p<0.05$). Only one of the 23 patients in the rhEPO arm was unable to donate 4 units or more compared with seven of 24 patients in the control arm. Likewise, in a randomized, placebo-controlled study of 50 women undergoing total hip replacement and having a basal hematocrit less than 40%, Mercuriali et al[83] found that patients receiving rhEPO donated significantly more autologous blood than those treated with a placebo (4.5 units compared with 2.8 units; $p<0.05$) and received significantly less allogeneic blood (0.4 unit per rhEPO-treated patient compared with 1.2 units per placebo-treated patient; $p<0.05$).

In order to study whether rhEPO can reduce the need for transfusion, a large, double-blind, randomized, placebo-controlled study was conducted at five centers in Canada involving patients undergoing elective hip replacement.[84] The 208 patients in this study were randomly assigned to one of three groups, each of which received daily subcutaneous injections of either rhEPO or a placebo beginning on day 10 preoperatively and continuing through the third postoperative day, for a total of 14 days. Group 1 received only a placebo, group 2 received rhEPO (300 U/kg daily) for the full 14 days, and group 3 was given a placebo for the first 5 days, followed by rhEPO for the next 9 days. All received ferrous sulfate 325 mg thrice daily.

In all cases, the decision to transfuse was in accordance with preestablished guidelines. A primary outcome event (transfusion and/or hemoglobin decline to below 8 g/dL) occurred least often in patients who received the full 14 days of rhEPO. Primary events occurred significantly less often in the rhEPO-treated groups (23% in the group receiving 14 days of rhEPO and 32% in those getting only 9 days compared with 46% in controls, $p = 0.003$). Transfusion rates were also significantly lower, with the lowest rate occurring in those treated with rhEPO for the longest time. Group 2 (14 days rhEPO) received a mean of 0.52 transfusion compared with 0.70 transfusion in group 3 (9 days rhEPO), and 1.14 transfusions in controls. No significant differences were seen in adverse effects, including deep vein thrombosis and hypertension, between the rhEPO-treated groups and those treated with iron alone.

A randomized, double-blind, placebo-controlled trial involving 116 patients donating autologous blood prior to surgery similarly showed that treatment with rhEPO resulted in increased red cell production in a dose-dependent fashion, but failed to demonstrate a benefit in reducing allogeneic blood exposure.[82] In this study, patients were given either a placebo or rhEPO in doses of 150, 300, or 600 U/kg intravenously at intervals of 3-4 days for a total of six doses during the 3-week study period. Placebo-treated patients produced approximately 400 mL of red blood cells, whereas those receiving 300 U/kg of rhEPO produced an additional 200 mL, and those treated with 600 U/kg produced 400 mL of additional red cells. Despite the fact that rhEPO treatment resulted in the production of red cell volumes equivalent to 1-2 additional units, the percentage of patients in each group who required allogeneic blood was not different (9% in each group), nor was the number of allogeneic units transfused per patient.

The Effect on Autologous Donation in the Anemic Patient

It has been suggested that rhEPO might be especially beneficial when used to facilitate blood donation by patients who are anemic at their first donation. A recent multicenter, randomized, double-blind, clinical trial involving 204 patients with baseline hematocrit of 39% or less who were scheduled for elective orthopedic surgery examined the impact of rhEPO on red cell collection and allogeneic blood exposure in patients with baseline anemia. Patients treated with rhEPO were able to collect more red cells, both in terms of volume and number of units, and required fewer allogeneic blood transfusions than did controls.[85] Patients in both arms were scheduled to donate every 3-4 days for 21 days if their hematocrit was at least 33%. At each visit, patients received either 600 U/kg intravenous rhEPO or a placebo. Patients in the rhEPO group collected on average 1.5 more units of red cells (4.5 units compared with 3.0 units) and 52% larger volumes of red cells (684 mL compared with 449 mL) than did control patients. Overall, 20% of the rhEPO-treated patients required allogeneic blood compared with 31% of the control patients (p = 0.09). With the application of logistic regression modeling, it became apparent that the risk of allogeneic blood transfusion was significantly affected not only by the type of surgery (p<0.001) and by the baseline hematocrit (p = 0.001) but also by rhEPO treatment (p = 0.025). When patients who required more than 6 units were excluded (ie, those patients who would have required allogeneic blood even if they had collected the maximum allowable volume of blood), allogeneic exposure rates in the rhEPO-treated group were less than half those seen with the controls (14% compared with 29%; p = 0.015). Subset analysis suggested that rhEPO may be most beneficial in mild to moderate anemia (hematocrit ≥ 33% or higher) when anticipated blood requirements are also moderate—3-6 units.

The Effect on the Postoperative Development of Anemia and on Hematocrit Recovery

Other studies have looked at the impact of rhEPO on the development of anemia following surgery and on the recovery time of hematocrit in postsurgical anemia and have found rhEPO to be beneficial in both of these settings.[86,87]

In a pilot study involving 10 patients undergoing distal gastrectomy, five were randomly selected to receive iron plus rhEPO (200 U/kg) for 7 days preoperatively and 14 days postoperatively, whereas five control patients received only iron.[86] Distal gastrectomy was chosen for the study because patients were unlikely to require transfusion, allowing the effect of rhEPO to be studied in the absence of blood transfusion. The rhEPO-treated arm showed no significant drop in packed cell volume on the first postoperative day, whereas the control arm showed a drop from 0.378 prior to surgery to 0.329 on day 1 (p<0.05). Likewise, hemoglobin concentrations were higher at both day 7 in the rhEPO group than in the control (13.7 g/dL vs 11.0 g/dL; p<0.05) and on day 10 (14.0 g/dL vs 10.8 g/dL). Only one patient required transfusion and that patient was in the control arm.

A study involving 40 Jehovah's Witnesses with severe postsurgical anemia (hematocrit <25%) who refused transfusion examined the role of rhEPO in stimulating the recovery of hematocrit in the immediate postoperative period.[87] Half of these patients received iron plus rhEPO in one of two dosing regimens, and the other 20 patients received iron alone. After one week, the rhEPO-treated group showed both a significantly higher hematocrit ($p<0.0005$) and a significantly greater rise in hematocrit ($p<0.005$). In week two, the increase in hematocrit was no longer significantly different ($p = 0.12$). The authors of this study conclude that, in the absence of rhEPO, the recovery of hematocrit in severely anemic postsurgical patients is characterized by a 1-week lag period and that the use of rhEPO can accelerate the recovery of hematocrit during this first postoperative week.

It is important to remember that intravenously administered rhEPO elicits a response in 3.5 days and results in the production of the equivalent of 1 unit of blood in approximately 7 days.[74,87,88] Thus, perioperative administration of rhEPO can be expected to replace only modest blood losses and would be of no value in the acute management of hemorrhage as the result of trauma.

Cost-Effectiveness

As with all therapeutic modalities in this age of cost-containment, any analysis of the utility of rhEPO therapy in the perioperative setting would not be complete without some cost-analysis data. Birkmeyer et al[89,90] have used decision analysis to look at the cost-effectiveness of PAD in the settings of coronary artery bypass grafting and of elective orthopedic surgery.[89,90] They concluded that PAD, at a cost generally in excess of $100,000 to $150,000 per quality-adjusted life year of life saved, is not cost effective in either of these settings. Even though they estimated PAD to cost less than $200 per patient, the cost-benefit of autologous donation may be marginal despite the lower risk of transfusion-associated complications. Thus, the denominator of the cost-divided-by-benefit equation was also low, which accounts for the high (unfavorable) cost-effectiveness estimates. Adding the cost of rhEPO, which was nearly $4000 (Canadian) for a 14-day course in the Canadian study, to the cost of PAD seems unlikely to improve these figures in all but the most extraordinary of cases, such as in patients with multiple red cell alloantibodies.

Summary

In summary, rhEPO has been shown to increase the volume of autologous blood that can be collected preoperatively, as well as to stimulate the recovery of hemoglobin and hematocrit when administered in the perioperative period. rhEPO may, therefore, be of particular use as an adjunct to PAD in patients who are small or anemic or for whom large volumes (4 or more units) of blood are needed. It may also have a role in allowing the collection of sufficient compatible blood for those patients who are known to have multiple red cell alloantibodies. In addition, rhEPO can be used effectively in patients such as Jehovah's Witnesses who refuse allogeneic blood transfusion. In fact, preparations of rhEPO are currently being developed that use stabilizers not derived from human blood components.

Conclusions

Erythropoietin is produced by the kidneys in response to increased transcription of the EPO gene induced by hypoxia and, thus, indirectly by anemia. It serves the vital function of stimulating erythropoiesis, thereby restoring oxygen delivery. Endogenous EPO production has been found to be inappropriately low in a number of anemic states, most notably in chronic renal failure; in the anemia of chronic disease; cancer; HIV infection; and in the anemia of prematurity.

Treatment with rhEPO has been evaluated in each of these settings, with mixed results. It appears to be highly effective in renal disease provided dialysis is adequate to remove circulating uremic toxins, in HIV patients with endogenous EPO levels less than 500 IU/L, and in certain subsets of cancer patients, most notably those with multiple myeloma. Its effectiveness in other cancer patients ranges from 40-70%, depending on the nature of concomitant therapy for the underlying malignancy. On the other hand, rhEPO is largely ineffective as a single agent in most myelodysplastic patients, although it may prove more effective when used in combination with G-CSF or when used as a single agent in patients with the refractory anemia FAB subtype and low (≤100 U/L) baseline endogenous EPO levels. And, while rhEPO may reduce red cell transfusion rates in very low-birth-weight infants with the anemia of prematurity, its cost-effectiveness remains in doubt. Cost-effectiveness is also an issue when rhEPO is used in the perioperative setting, either to enhance the collection of autologous blood for use at surgery or as a means of stimulating the recovery of hematocrit in the immediate postoperative period.

References

1. Romanowski RR, Sytkowski AJ. The molecular structure of human erythropoietin. Hematol Oncol Clin North Am 1994;8:885-94.
2. McGuire MJ, Spivak JL. Erythropoiesis. In: Anderson KC, Ness PM, eds. Scientific basis of transfusion medicine: Implications for clinical practice. Philadelphia, PA: W. B. Saunders Company, 1994:1-16.
3. Spivak JL. The clinical physiology of erythropoietin. Semin Hematol 1993;30:2-11.

4. Semenza GL. Regulation of erythropoietin production: New insights into molecular mechanisms of oxygen homeostasis. Hematol Oncol Clin North Am 1994;8:863-84.
5. Sawyer ST, Penta K. Erythropoietin cell biology. Hematol Oncol Clin North Am 1994;8:895-911.
6. Eschbach JW, Egrie JC, Downing MR, et al. Correction of the anemia of end-stage renal disease with recombinant human erythropoietin: Results of a combined phase I and II clinical trial. N Engl J Med 1987;316:73-8.
7. Eschbach JW, Abdulhadi MH, Browne JK, et al. Recombinant human erythropoietin in anemic patients with end-stage renal diseases: Results of a phase III multicenter clinical trial. Ann Intern Med 1989; 111:992-1000.
8. Gimenez LF, Scheel PJ. Clinical application of recombinant erythropoietin in renal dialysis patients. Hematol Oncol Clin North Am 1994;8:913-26.
9. Lim VS, DeGowin RL, Zavala D, et al. Recombinant human erythropoietin treatment in pre-dialysis patients: A double-blind placebo-controlled trial. Ann Intern Med 1989;110;108-14.
10. Ad Hoc Committee for the National Kidney Foundation. NKF position paper: Statement on the clinical use of recombinant erythropoietin in anemia of end-stage renal disease. Am J Kidney Dis 1989;14:163-9.
11. The US Recombinant Human Erythropoietin Predialysis Study Group. Double-blind, placebo-controlled study of the therapeutic use of recombinant human erythropoietin for anemia associated with chronic renal failure in predialysis patients. Am J Kidney Dis 1991;18:50-9.
12. Piraino B, Johnston JR. The use of subcutaneous erythropoietin in CAPD patients. Clin Nephrol 1990;33:200-2.
13. Taylor JE, Belch JJF, Fleming LW, et al. Erythropoietin response and route of administration. Clin Nephrol 1994;41:297-302.
14. Stone WJ, Graber SE, Krantz SB, et al. Treatment of anemia of predialysis patients with recombinant human erythropoietin: A randomized, placebo-controlled trial. Am J Med Sci 1988;296:171-9.
15. Kleinman KS, Schweitzer SU, Perdue ST, et al. The use of recombinant human erythropoietin in the correction of anemia in predialysis patients and its effect on renal function: A double-blind, placebo controlled trial. Am J Kidney Dis 1989;14:486-95.
16. Klahr S. Anemia, dialysis, and dollars. N Engl J Med 1996;334:461-3.
17. Sisk JE, Gianfrancesco FD, Coster JM. Recombinant erythropoietin and medicare payment. JAMA 1991;266:247-52.

18. Ifudu O, Feldman J, Friedman EA. The intensity of hemodialysis and the response to erythropoietin in patients with end-stage renal disease. N Engl J Med 1996;334:420-5.
19. Goodnough LT, Strasburg D, Riddell J, et al. Has recombinant erythropoietin therapy minimized red cell transfusions in hemodialysis patients? Clin Nephrol 1994;41:303-7.
20. Nelson DA, Davey FR. Erythrocytic disorders. In: Henry JB, ed. Clinical diagnosis and management by laboratory methods. 18th ed. Philadelphia, PA: W. B. Saunders Company, 1991:670.
21. Means RT, Krantz SB. Progress in understanding the pathogenesis of the anemia of chronic disease. Blood 1992;80:1639-47.
22. Miller CB, Jones RJ, Piantadosi S, et al. Decreased erythropoietin response in patients with the anemia of cancer. N Engl J Med 1990;322:1689-92.
23. Baer AN, Dessypris EN, Goldwasser E, Krantz SB. Blunted erythropoietin response to anaemia in rheumatoid arthritis. Br J Haematol 1987;66:559-64.
24. Means RT. Clinical application of recombinant erythropoietin in the anemia of chronic disease. Hematol Oncol Clin North Am 1994; 8:933-44.
25. Cash JM, Sears DA. The anemia of chronic disease: Spectrum of associated diseases in a series of unselected hospitalized patients. Am J Med 1989;87:638-44.
26. Means RT, Olsen NJ, Krantz SB, et al. Treatment of the anemia of rheumatoid arthritis with recombinant human erythropoietin: Clinical and in vitro studies. Arthritis Rheum 1989;32:638-42.
27. Pincus T, Olsen NJ, Wolfe F, et al. Multicenter study of recombinant human erythropoietin in correction of anemia in rheumatoid arthritis. Am J Med 1990;89:161-8.
28. Thompson FL, Powers JS, Graber SE, Krantz SB. Use of recombinant human erythropoietin to enhance autologous blood donation in a patient with multiple red cell allo-antibodies and the anemia of chronic disease. Am J Med 1991;90:398-400.
29. Case DC, Bukowski RM, Cary RW, et al. Recombinant human erythropoietin therapy for anemic cancer patients on combination chemotherapy. J Natl Cancer Inst 1993;85:801-6.
30. Spivak JL, Barnes DC, Fuch E, Quinn TC. Serum immunoreactive erythropoietin in HIV-infected patients. JAMA 1989;261;3104-7.
31. Zon LI, Arkin C, Groopman JE. Haematologic manifestations of the human immune deficiency virus (HIV). Br J Haematol 1987;66:251-6.

32. Henry DH, Beall GN, Benson CA, et al. Recombinant human erythropoietin in the treatment of anemia associated with human immunodeficiency virus (HIV) infection and zidovudine therapy: Overview of four clinical trials. Ann Intern Med 1992;117:739-48.
33. Richman DD, Fischl MA, Grieco MH, et al. The toxicity of azidothymidine (AZT) in the treatment of patients with AIDS and AIDS-related complex: A double-blind, placebo-controlled trial. N Engl J Med 1987;317:192-7.
34. Phair JP, Abels RI, McNeill MV, Sullivan DJ. Recombinant human erythropoietin treatment: Investigational new drug protocol for the anemia of the acquired immunodeficiency syndrome: Overall results. Arch Intern Med 1993;153:2669-75.
35. Perno CF, Cooney DA, Gao WY, et al. Effects of bone marrow stimulatory cytokines on human immunodeficiency virus replication and the antiviral activity of dideoxynucleosides in cultures of monocyte/macrophages. Blood 1992;80:995-1003.
36. Fischl M, Galpin JE, Levine JD, et al. Recombinant human erythropoietin for patients with AIDS treated with zidovudine. N Engl J Med 1990;322:1488-93.
37. Glaspy JA, Chap L. The clinical application of recombinant erythropoietin in the HIV-infected patient. Hematol Oncol Clin North Am 1994;8:945-59.
38. Miles SA, Mitsuyasu RT, Moreno J, et al. Combined therapy with recombinant granulocyte colony-stimulating factor and erythropoietin decreases hematologic toxicity from zidovudine. Blood 1991;77: 2109-17.
39. Ludwig H, Fritz E, Kotzmann H, et al. Erythropoietin treatment of anemia associated with multiple myeloma. N Engl J Med 1990;322: 1693-9.
40. Henry DH. Clinical application of recombinant erythropoietin in anemic cancer patients. Hematol Oncol Clin North Am 1994;8:961-73.
41. Oster W, Herrmann F, Gamm H, et al. Erythropoietin for the treatment of anemia of malignancy associated with neoplastic bone marrow infiltration. J Clin Oncol 1990;8:956-62.
42. Platanais LC, Miller CB, Mick R, et al. Treatment of chemotherapy-induced anemia with recombinant human erythropoietin in cancer patients. J Clin Oncol 1991;9:2021-6.
43. Henry DH, Abels RI. Recombinant human erythropoietin in the treatment of cancer and chemotherapy-induced anemia: Results of double-blind and open-label follow-up studies. Semin Oncol 1994;21:21-8.

44. Henry D, Abels R, Larholt K. Prediction of response to recombinant human erythropoietin (r-Hu EPO/Epoetin-α) therapy in cancer patients. Blood 1995;85:1676-8.
45. Ludwig H, Fritz E, Leitgeb C, et al. Prediction of response to erythropoietin treatment in chronic anemia of cancer. Blood 1994;84:1056-63.
46. Barlogie B. Treatment of the anemia of multiple myeloma: The role of recombinant human erythropoietin. Semin Hematol 1993;30:25-7.
47. Mittelman M, Lessin LS. Clinical application of recombinant erythropoietin in myelodysplasia. Hematol Oncol Clin North Am 1994;8: 993-1009.
48. Greenberg PL. Use of recombinant human erythropoietin to treat the anemia of myelodysplastic syndromes. Semin Hematol 1993;30:22-4.
49. Negrin RS, Stein R, Vardiman J, et al. Treatment of the anemia of myelodysplastic syndromes using recombinant human granulocyte-stimulating factor in combination with erythropoietin. Blood 1993; 82:737-43.
50. Rose EH, Abels RI, Nelson RA, et al. The use of r-HuEpo in the treatment of anaemia related to myelodysplasia (MDS). Br J Haematol 1995;89:831-7.
51. Beguin Y, Clemons GK, Oris R, Fillet G. Circulating erythropoietin levels after bone marrow transplantation: Inappropriate response to anemia in allogeneic transplants. Blood 1991;77:868-73.
52. Ireland RM, Atkinson K, Concannon A, et al. Serum erythropoietin changes in autologous and allogeneic bone marrow transplant patients. Br J Haematol 1990;76:128-34.
53. Locatelli F, Zecca M, Pedrazzoli P, et al. Use of recombinant human erythropoietin after bone marrow transplantation in pediatric patients with leukemia: Effect on erythroid repopulation in autologous versus allogeneic transplants. Bone Marrow Transplant 1994;13:403-10.
54. Biggs JC, Atkinson KA, Booker V, et al. Prospective randomised double-blind trial of the in vivo use of recombinant human erythropoietin in bone marrow transplantation from HLA-identical sibling donors. Bone Marrow Transplant 1995;15:129-34.
55. Klaesson S. Ringden O, Ljungman P, et al. Reduced blood transfusions requirements after allogeneic bone marrow transplantation: Results of a randomised, double-blind study with high-dose erythropoietin. Bone Marrow Transplant 1994;13:397-402.
56. Ayash LJ, Elias A, Hunt M, et al. Recombinant human erythropoietin for the treatment of the anaemia associated with autologous bone marrow transplantation. Br J Haematol 1994;87:153-61.

57. Miller CB, Mills S, Barnett AG, Beveridge RA, Jones RJ. A randomized trial of recombinant human erythropoietin (rHuEPO) after purged autologous bone marrow transplant (BMT) (abstract). Blood 1993;82: 285a.
58. Miller AM, Dempsey H, Weiner RS, et al. Recombinant human erythropoietin does not promote "stem-cell steal" following autologous bone marrow transplant (abstract). Blood 1993;82:638a.
59. Miller CB, Mills S. Erythropoietin after bone marrow transplantation. Hematol Oncol Clin North Am 1994;8:975-92.
60. Fain J, Hilsenrath P, Widness J, et al. A cost analysis comparing erythropoietin and red cell transfusions in the treatment of anemia of prematurity. Transfusion 1995;35:936-43.
61. Strauss RG. Erythropoietin in the pathogenesis and treatment of neonatal anemia. Transfusion 1995;35:68-73.
62. Shannon KM, Keith JF, Mentzer WC, et al. Recombinant human erythropoietin stimulates erythropoiesis and reduces erythrocyte transfusions in very low birth weight preterm infants. Pediatrics 1995;95:1-8.
63. Shannon KM, Mentzer WC, Abels RI, et al. Recombinant human erythropoietin in the anemia of prematurity: Results of a placebo-controlled pilot study. J Pediatr 1991;118:949-55.
64. Meyer MP, Meyer JH, Commerford A, et al. Recombinant human erythropoietin in the treatment of the anemia of prematurity: Results of a double-blind, placebo-controlled study. Pediatrics 1994; 93:918-23.
65. Soubasi V, Kremenopoulos G, Diamanti E, et al. Follow-up of very low birth weight infants after erythropoietin treatment to prevent anemia of prematurity. J Pediatr 1995;127:291-7.
66. Ohls RK, Osborne KA, Christensen RD. Efficacy and cost analysis of treating very low birth weight infants with erythropoietin during their first two weeks of life: A randomized, placebo-controlled trial. J Pediatr 1995;126:421-6.
67. Maier RF, Obladen M, Scigalla P, et al. The effect of epoietin beta (recombinant human erythropoietin) on the need for transfusion in very-low-birth-weight infants. N Engl J Med 1994;330:1173-8.
68. Carnielli V, Montini G, Da Riol R, et al. Effect of high doses of human recombinant erythropoietin on the need for blood transfusions in preterm infants. J Pediatr 1992;121:98-102.
69. Hume H, Bard H. Small volume red blood cell transfusions for neonatal patients. Transfus Med Rev 1995;9:187-99.

70. Goodnough LT, Price TH, Rudnick S, Soegiarso RW. Preoperative red cell production in patients undergoing aggressive autologous blood phlebotomy with and without erythropoietin therapy. Transfusion 1992;32:441-5.
71. Liu EA, Mannino FL, Lane TA. Prospective, randomized trial of the safety and efficacy of a limited donor exposure transfusion program for premature neonates. J Pediatr 1994;125:92-6.
72. Emmerson AJB, Coles HJ, Pearson TC. Double blind trial of recombinant human erythropoietin in preterm infants. Arch Dis Child 1993; 68:291-6.
73. Wilimas JA, Crist WM. Erythropoietin—not yet a standard treatment for anemia of prematurity. Pediatrics 1995;95:9-10.
74. Goodnough LT. Clinical application of recombinant erythropoietin in the perioperative period. Hematol Oncol Clin North Am 1994;8: 1011-20.
75. Goodnough LT, Shafron D, Marcus RE. The impact of preoperative autologous blood donation on orthopaedic surgical practice. Vox Sang 1990;59:65-9.
76. Mercuriali F, Adamson JW. Recombinant human erythropoietin enhances blood donation for autologous use and reduces exposure to homologous blood during elective surgery. Semin Hematol 1993;30:17-21.
77. Goodnough LT, Vizmeg K, Verbrugge D. The impact of autologous blood ordering and blood procurement practices on allogeneic blood exposure in elective orthopedic surgery patients. Am J Clin Pathol 1994;101:354-7.
78. Goodnough LT, Brittenham GM. Limitations of the erythropoietic response to serial phlebotomy: Implications for autologous blood donor programs. J Lab Clin Med 1990;115:28-35.
79. Tasaki T, Ohto H, Noguchi M, et al. Iron and erythropoietin measurement in autologous blood donors with anemia: Implications for management. Transfusion 1994;34:337-43.
80. Goodnough LT, Rudnick S, Price TH, et al. Increased preoperative collection of autologous blood with recombinant human erythropoietin therapy. N Engl J Med 1989;321:1163-8.
81. Tasaki T, Ohto J, Hashimoto C, et al. Recombinant human erythropoietin for autologous blood donation: Effects on perioperative red-blood-cell and serum erythropoietin production. Lancet 1992;339: 773-5.
82. Goodnough LT, Price TH, Friedman KD, et al. A phase III trial of recombinant human erythropoietin therapy in nonanemic orthopedic

patients subjected to aggressive removal of blood for autologous use: Dose, response, toxicity and efficacy. Transfusion 1994;34:66-71.

83. Mercuriali F, Zanella A, Barosi G, et al. Use of erythropoietin to increase the volume of autologous blood donated by orthopedic patients. Transfusion 1993;33:55-60.
84. Canadian Orthopedic Perioperative Erythropoietin Study Group. Effectiveness of perioperative recombinant human erythropoietin in elective hip replacement. Lancet 1993;341:1227-32.
85. Price TH, Goodnough LT, Vogler WR, et al. The effect of recombinant human erythropoietin on the efficacy of autologous blood donation in patients with low hematocrits: A multicenter, randomized, double-blind, controlled trial. Transfusion 1996;36:29-36.
86. Tsuji Y, Kambayashi JI, Shiba E, et al. Effect of recombinant human erythropoietin on anaemia after gastrectomy: A pilot study. Eur J Surg 1995;161:29-33.
87. Atabek U, Alvarez R, Pello MJ, et al. Erythropoietin accelerates hematocrit recovery in post-surgical anemia. Am Surg 1995;61:74-7.
88. AuBuchon JP. Minimizing donor exposure in hemotherapy. Arch Pathol Lab Med 1994;118:380-91.
89. Birkmeyer JD, AuBuchon JP, Littenberg B, et al. Cost-effectiveness of preoperative autologous donation in coronary artery bypass grafting. Ann Thorac Surg 1994;57:161-9.
90. Birkmeyer JD, Goodnough LT, AuBuchon JP, et al. The cost-effectiveness of preoperative autologous blood donation for total hip and knee replacement. Transfusion 1993;33:544-51.

In: Davenport RD, Snyder EL, eds.
Cytokines in Transfusion Medicine: A Primer
Bethesda, MD: AABB Press, 1997

6

Leukocyte Growth Factors in Granulocyte and Allogeneic Peripheral Blood Progenitor Cell Donors

DAVID F. STRONCEK, MD, AND
SUSAN F. LEITMAN, MD

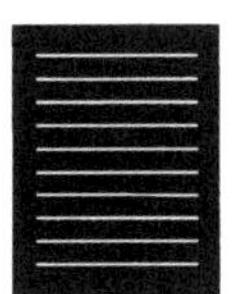

GRANULOCYTE COLONY-STIMULATING FACTOR (G-CSF) and granulocyte-macrophage colony-stimulating factor (GM-CSF), two of the most widely used growth factors in clinical medicine, are among the few growth factors that are given to healthy donors. Both G-CSF and GM-CSF can be used to mobilize hematopoietic progenitor cells for autologous and allogeneic transplantation. G-CSF is more effective at mobilizing hematopoietic progeni-

David F. Stroncek, MD, Chief, Laboratory Services Section; and Susan F. Leitman, MD, Chief, Blood Services, and Deputy Chief, Department of Transfusion Medicine, Warren G. Magnuson Clinical Center, National Institutes of Health, Bethesda, Maryland

tors and neutrophils and is better tolerated by donors. Therefore, when peripheral blood progenitor cells (PBPCs) are collected from healthy donors, G-CSF is almost always preferred. At many transplant centers, PBPCs collected by apheresis from healthy donors who are given G-CSF are being used in place of marrow for transplants involving HLA-matched siblings.[1-7] G-CSF is also becoming the standard agent for increasing granulocyte counts in healthy volunteer granulocyte donors.[8-11]

Both G-CSF and GM-CSF have been used in a number of other clinical settings,[12-15] for example, to decrease the period of neutropenia in patients treated with myeloablative chemotherapy or in patients who have received marrow transplants. They have also been used to treat patients with congenital or immune-mediated neutropenia, cyclic neutropenia, aplastic anemia, and acquired immune deficiency syndrome (AIDS)-related neutropenia. This chapter reviews the use of G-CSF and GM-CSF in healthy donors for the purpose of mobilizing PBPCs for allogeneic transplantation and granulocytes for transfusion.

Granulocyte- and PBPC-Mobilizing Agents

G-CSF

G-CSF is a 24-25 kDa glycoprotein that is produced by monocytes, macrophages, endothelial cells, fibroblasts, and mesothelial cells.[12-14] It has 174 amino acids, is variably glycosylated, and is encoded by a single gene on chromosome 17q11-22. Two forms of human recombinant G-CSF are currently manufactured: lenograstim, which is glycosylated, and filgrastim, which is not. Only filgrastim is available in the United States at this time. Filgrastim can be given either subcutaneously or intravenously. Its half-life is 3.5 hours.

GM-CSF

Human GM-CSF is a 22 kDa glycoprotein[12,16] with 127 amino acids. The gene that encodes GM-CSF has 2.5 kilobases and is located on chromosome 5q21-32. GM-CSF is produced by T lymphocytes, macrophages, mast cells, endothelial cells, and certain fibroblasts. Serum levels of human recombinant GM-CSF, sargramostim, peak 2-3 hours after subcutaneous injection and its half-life is about 2-3 hours.

The Mobilization of Granulocytes and Hematopoietic Progenitors

G-CSF

The Mobilization of Granulocytes

In healthy donors, neutrophils are mobilized by a single injection of G-CSF. Within 30 minutes of a G-CSF injection, neutrophils become activated and their expression of Fc-γ-receptor III (FcγRIII, CD16), CD13, CD45, CD67, and CD11b increases.[17] The neutrophil counts fall during the first 30 minutes following the injection, but by 4 hours after the injection neutrophil counts begin to increase; the expression of CD13, CD45, CD11b, and CD67 returns to pre-G-CSF levels; the expression of FcγRIII falls below pre-G-CSF levels; and the expression of CD14 and FcγRI (CD64) increases. Within 12 hours after the injection of 300 μg of G-CSF to a healthy adult, neutrophil counts peak at about 20×10^9 cells/L, the expression of FcγRIII remains decreased, and the expression of FcγRI and CD14 remains increased.[17] The neutrophil counts remain increased at 15 to 20×10^9/L at 24 hours after the injection, but then gradually return to normal at 72 hours after the injection.

If repeated daily doses of G-CSF are given, neutrophil counts increase further for 2-3 more days and then reach a plateau (Fig 6-1).[18] Neutrophil counts that are measured each morning are at a plateau after three or four injections, although, when G-CSF is given daily as a single morning dose, the neutrophil counts fall within 1 hour of each injection, increase over the next 12 hours and then return to the preinjection level. The neutrophil counts measured at 12 hours after each injection are approximately twice the pre-G-CSF counts.[19]

The donor's white blood cell (WBC) count can rise as high as 80×10^9 cells/L when 10 μg/kg of G-CSF is given daily. These elevated leukocyte counts have not been reported to cause symptoms in healthy donors, but some centers reduce the G-CSF dose if the counts exceed 50-70 $\times 10^9$ cells/L.[15] The magnitude of the elevation on the sixth day is dose-dependent, at least up to doses of 7.5 mg/kg/day (Fig 6-1). The number of neutrophils that are mobilized is independent of the donor's age even up to 70-80 years of age.[19]

Other circulating blood cells are affected variably by G-CSF administration. In healthy donors, monocyte and lymphocyte counts are slightly elevated by G-CSF, but eosinophil and basophil counts usually do not change during the administration of G-CSF.[12,13,18] Hemoglobin, hematocrit, and re-

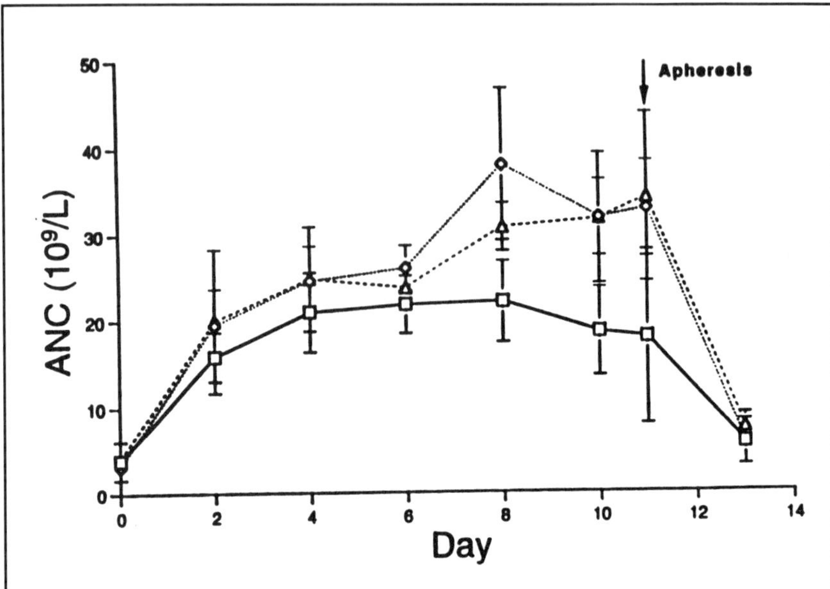

Figure 6-1. Neutrophil counts in healthy donors who were given G-CSF. G-CSF 2 (-□-, n = 6), 5 (-◊-, n =7), or 7.5 (-△-, n =2) µg/kg was given subcutaneously daily for 10 days (days 1 - 10) and PBPCs were collected once (day 11, arrow). The values represent the mean ± SD. ANC = absolute neutrophil count. (Used with permission from Stroncek et al.[18])

ticulocyte counts do not change during the G-CSF course, but if G-CSF is given for more than 4 or 5 days, the donors' platelet counts fall by 22% after 9 days and 28% after 10 days.[20]

G-CSF increases the cellularity of the marrow and the total number of neutrophils that are produced.[21] In addition, G-CSF decreases the transit time of the neutrophils through the marrow. Normally, it takes 4 or 5 days for cells to progress from myeloid progenitors to circulating neutrophils, but when G-CSF is given, the transit time of neutrophils through the marrow is reduced to only 1 day.[21] Once they are released from the marrow, the circulating half-life of G-CSF-mobilized neutrophils is approximately 24 hours compared with the 8-hour half-life reported for nonmobilized cells.[21]

The Function of G-CSF-Mobilized Granulocytes

While a single dose of G-CSF has a dramatic effect on the number of granulocytes that can be collected, this cytokine modifies several quantitative characteristics of granulocytes as well. In vitro studies have found that G-CSF enhances several neutrophil functions including superoxide production, degranulation, phagocytosis, and the migration of neutrophils across unstimulated endothelium.[22-24] However, G-CSF-mobilized neutrophils are deficient in two important neutrophil antigens: FcγRIII (CD16) and L-selectin (CD62L). The lack of FcγRIII expression by G-CSF-mobilized granulocytes probably does not affect the function of these cells significantly. Subjects with a congenital deficiency of FcγRIII have not been found to be at an increased risk for bacterial or fungal infection.[25] Lack of expression of L-selectin, on the other hand, may have a significant detrimental effect.

L-selectin is an important mediator of interactions between neutrophils and endothelial cells, and an animal model suggests that neutrophils lacking L-selectin may be less able to migrate into areas of inflammation.[26] However, paradoxically, the reduction of L-selectin expression could make the transfusion of these neutrophils more effective rather than less effective. Preliminary studies have found that the in-vivo half-life of G-CSF-mobilized granulocytes is significantly longer than that of granulocytes mobilized with only dexamethasone,[8-11] and the prolonged circulation may partly be due to the decrease in L-selectin expression.

Ordinarily, following granulocyte transfusions, most of the transfused cells become trapped transiently in lungs.[27] If this pulmonary sequestration of neutrophils is mediated by L-selectin, then neutrophils from G-CSF-stimulated donors might have a greater and a more immediate posttransfusion intravascular recovery and be less likely to cause the pulmonary reactions that are well recognized after some infusions. Because G-CSF effects several changes in granulocyte function and membrane antigen expression, it is difficult to predict how effective the transfusion of G-CSF-mobilized granulocytes will be in treating infections.

The Mobilization of Hematopoietic Progenitor Cells

The mobilization of hematopoietic progenitor cells in healthy donors differs from the mobilization of granulocytes in two important ways: 1) there is an increase in progenitor cells only after two or three daily injections of G-CSF[18,28-35] and 2) the increase is only temporary.[18,33] The circulating concentrations of colony-forming cells (CFCs), long-term culture-initiating cells (LT-CICs), and CD34+ cells are all increased by G-CSF, but because CD34+ cells are the most readily quantitated, the kinetics of CD34+ cell mobilization have been studied best.

During the first 48 hours of daily G-CSF administration, there is no increase in the number of circulating CD34+ cells, but on the third day, the CD34+ cell count begins to increase and continues to increase until a maximum is reached on the fifth or sixth day. The day of the peak CD34+ cell number varies among individuals, but the maximum almost always occurs on the fifth or sixth day.[36] After the sixth day, the CD34+ cell count falls even if daily G-CSF injections are continued (Fig 6-2).[18] On the eighth day, the CD34+ cell counts are significantly lower than the peak counts; on the tenth day the counts fall to one-third of the peak counts; and on the eleventh day, the counts fall to only one-fourth of the peak counts.[18] Continued administration of a growth factor does not result in a further rise in CD34+ cells.

The magnitude of the increase in CD34+ cell counts is dependent on the dose of G-CSF, at least to daily doses of 10 μg/kg. When a healthy donor is given daily subcutaneous injections of G-CSF (10 μg/kg), the

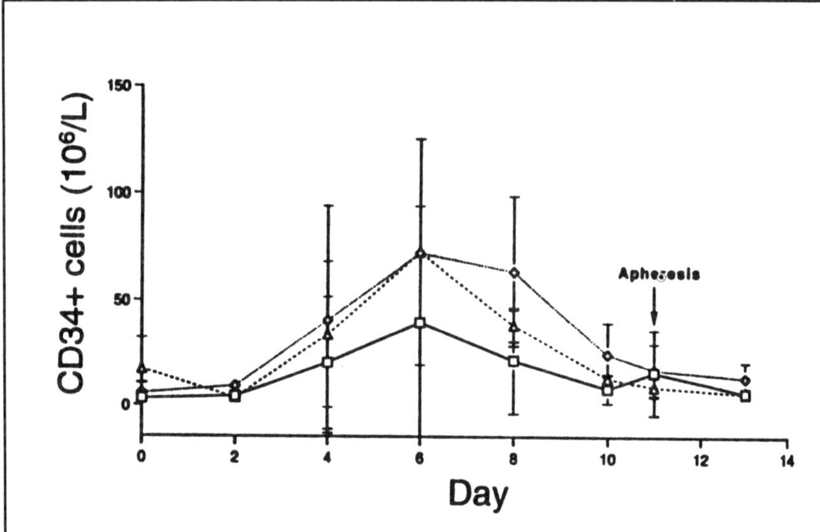

Figure 6-2. Circulating CD34+ cell counts in healthy donors who were given G-CSF. G-CSF 2 (-□-, n = 6), 5 (-◇-, n = 7), or 7.5 (-△-, n = 2) μg/kg G-CSF was given subcutaneously daily for 10 days (days 1 - 10) and PBPCs were collected once (day 11, arrow). The values represent the mean ± SD. (Used with permission from Stroncek et al.[18])

CD34+ cell count increases on the sixth day by 20- to 30-fold to $76 \pm 61 \times 10^6$ cells/L.[18] Additional mobilization of CD34+ cells may occur with G-CSF doses greater than 10 μg/kg/day, but published, dose-response studies have not evaluated enough donors to show a statistically significant increase in CD34+ cell mobilization by doses above 10 μg/kg/day.[32]

When G-CSF is used to mobilize hematopoietic progenitor cells, it is usually given as a daily morning injection of 5-16 μg/kg. At some centers, G-CSF is given twice daily. One study that compared the effects of giving 12 μg/kg/day of G-CSF to donors as a single dose with giving 6 μg/kg to donors twice daily suggests that the twice-daily dose is more effective at mobilizing CD34+ cells.[37] However, it is much more convenient to administer the drug only once per day.

The number of CD34+ cells that are mobilized varies markedly among individuals. When 5-10 μg/kg/day is given to donors for 5 days, the circulating CD34+ cell counts on the sixth day range from 8.1×10^6 cells/L to 155.3×10^6 cells/L.[38] In addition to being affected by the G-CSF dose per kg, the number of cells that are mobilized correlates with the weight of the donor and weakly with the number of CD34+ cells in the donor's circulation prior to the administration of G-CSF.[38]

The Types of Hematopoietic Cells Mobilized

The CD34+ cells in the blood and the marrow can be divided into fractions or subpopulations on the basis of their expression of other membrane antigens. The quantities of the different subpopulations of CD34+ cells present in the blood of healthy donors who are given G-CSF differ from the quantities of the subpopulations of CD34+ cells that are normally present in the marrow. Compared with the CD34+ cells found in the marrow, the CD34+ cells that are present in the blood of healthy donors who are given G-CSF are more likely to be committed to the myeloid lineage and less likely to be committed to the lymphoid lineage. G-CSF-mobilized CD34+ cells are less likely to express the T-cell marker CD2 and the B-cell markers CD10, CD19, and CD20 but are more likely to express myeloid-associated surface molecules CD13, CD14, CD15, and CD33.[33,39-41] Primitive CD34+ cells are present in about the same proportions in mobilized blood and marrow. A more primitive fraction of CD34+ cells, cells that do not express CD38 or HLA-DR antigens, are either slightly decreased or the same in the mobilized blood of healthy donors who are given G-CSF as they are in normal marrow.[39-42]

The number of hematopoietic cells in the blood as quantitated by progenitor culture assays is also increased several-fold by G-CSF. In healthy donors, G-CSF increases the blood concentration of burst-forming unit–erythroid (BFU-E), colony-forming unit–granulocyte-macrophage (CFU-GM), CFU-Mix, and CD34+ cells to a similar degree, 20- to 30-fold.[43] However, G-CSF increases the blood concentration of long-term colony-initiating cells (LTC-ICs) seven-fold more than any of the other progenitors.[42]

However, the LTC-ICs mobilized by G-CSF differ from the LTC-ICs in the marrow. In marrow, most of the LTC-ICs are found in the CD34+ CD38– cell subpopulation, and these CD34+ CD38– LTC-ICs can be maintained in culture for 8 weeks or longer, indicating that they are very primitive progenitors. In contrast, in the blood of healthy donors who are given G-CSF, most of the LTC-ICs are present in a subpopulation of cells that express both CD34 and CD38 antigens, CD34+ CD38+ cells.[43] The CD34+ CD38+ LTC-ICs subpopulation of cells that are present in the blood after G-CSF stimulation are capable of sustaining hematopoiesis for 5, but not 8, weeks and, hence, are a more differentiated progenitor. During G-CSF mobilization the number of LTC-ICs in the blood that are found in the more primitive CD34+ CD38– cell subpopulation is increased, but to a much lesser degree than the CD34+ CD38+ LTC-IC subpopulation.[43] The CD34+ CD38– LTC-IC subpopulation in the blood of G-CSF-stimulated donors is similar to the bone marrow CD34+ CD38– subpopulation in that it can sustain hematopoiesis in culture for 8 weeks.

After 5 days of administration of G-CSF to healthy donors, most of the increase in the total number of circulating LTC-ICs is in the more committed CD34+ CD38+ progenitor subpopulation, which can be sustained in culture for only 5 weeks. While long-term durable hematopoietic engraftment of patients is likely provided by the primitive CD34+ CD38– progenitors, and not by the more committed CD34+ CD38+ progenitors, the large number of committed progenitors that are mobilized and present in the PBPCs is likely responsible for the more rapid recovery of neutrophil and platelet counts in patients who receive G-CSF-mobilized PBPC transplantation.

The Mechanisms of the Mobilization of Hematopoietic Cells

When G-CSF is administered to donors for 5 days, the concentrations of CFCs, LT-CICs, and CD34+ cells in the blood increase several-fold, but no significant increase occurs in the number of these progenitors in the marrow.[42] These results suggest that the mobilization of progenitor cells is not due to the crowding out of hematopoietic cells from the marrow. Rather, progenitor cells are probably mobilized by the release of cells from the marrow or the selective expansion of a subpopulation of cells that may be more likely to be present in the blood rather than the marrow.

Animal models suggest that the integrin adhesion receptor VLA-4, or α_4, plays an important role in the mobilization of hematopoietic progenitors. The treatment of nonhuman primates with a monoclonal antibody to α_4 selectively mobilizes progenitors into the blood at concentrations of 200 times baseline.[44]

A study of healthy donors who were given G-CSF supports the idea that a selected subpopulation of cells is expanded or released from the marrow.[42] In this study, healthy donors were given 10 μg/kg of G-CSF for 5 days. Their blood and marrow progenitors were analyzed, and adherence to marrow at stromal cells was compared before and after the administration of G-CSF. Progenitor cells in the blood were less adherent to marrow stroma than were progenitors in the marrow before G-CSF administration. After the 5-day course of G-CSF, the blood progenitors remained less adherent to bone marrow stroma than did the marrow progenitors.

This decrease in adherence of blood progenitors to bone marrow stroma was associated with a decrease in the expression of $\alpha_4\beta_1$ integrin, VLA-4, on circulating CD34+ cells compared with CD34+ cells in the marrow. The α_4 integrin expression on circulating CD34+ cells was less than the expression on marrow CD34+ cells both before and after G-CSF was given.

While the blood progenitors express less α_4 integrin, it does not appear that G-CSF directly down-regulates the expression of α_4 on marrow progenitors. When marrow progenitors that were collected prior to the administration of G-CSF were incubated in vitro with G-CSF, their expression of α_4 and their adhesion to marrow stroma did not decrease, but actually increased.[42]

These results suggest that a population of progenitor cells may normally circulate in the blood because they have a decreased expression of α_4 integrin and decreased adherence to marrow stroma. When G-CSF is administered, a subpopulation of progenitor cells that are less likely to express α_4 and more likely to be in the blood is selectively expanded or, alternatively, G-CSF down-regulates the expression of α_4 on marrow progenitors and releases them from the marrow. If G-CSF does induce a decrease in the expression of α_4 on marrow progenitors, these effects must be indirect because the addition of G-CSF to marrow progenitors in culture causes the expression of α_4 to increase.

GM-CSF

The Mobilization of Granulocytes

When a single dose of GM-CSF is given to healthy donors, their neutrophil and monocyte counts fall within 15 minutes.[24] The counts reach a nadir of less than 25% of the preinfusion counts 30 minutes after the injection. GM-

CSF causes a more prolonged neutropenia than G-CSF. After G-CSF is given, the counts fall, but return to normal within 60 minutes. In contrast, when GM-CSF is given, the counts remain below the preinfusion level for more than 120 minutes.[24]

When daily subcutaneous GM-CSF injections are given to donors, the number of circulating neutrophils increases but not to the same degree as with G-CSF.[45,46] Lane and colleagues[45] compared WBC and neutrophil counts in five healthy donors who were given 10 μg/kg/day of GM-CSF or 10 μg/kg/day of G-CSF for 4 days. In the subjects given G-CSF, WBC counts increased to 20 to 30 $\times$ 10^9 cells/L 24 hours after the first dose, but only increased to 5 to 10 $\times$ 10^9 cells/L in those who were given GM-CSF. After 4 days, the mean WBC was near 40 $\times$ 10^9 cells/L in the subjects who were given G-CSF, but was only 15 $\times$ 10^9 cells/L in subjects who were given GM-CSF. In a similar study, Fritsch and colleagues[46] found that after 5 days of administering 5 μg/kg of G-CSF to healthy donors, the WBC count increased to 33.0 $\pm$ 6.5 $\times$ 10^9 cells/L, but after five days of 5 μg/kg of GM-CSF, the WBC count increased to 15.2 $\pm$ 3.6 $\times$ 10^9 cells/L. In addition to mobilizing neutrophils, GM-CSF induces a dose-related increase in the monocyte and eosinophil count.[16]

GM-CSF increases the number of neutrophil and eosinophil precursors in the marrow and increases the production of neutrophils by 50%. In contrast to G-CSF, GM-CSF has no effect on the 4- to 5-day transit time of neutrophils through the marrow. GM-CSF does have a marked effect on the half-life of neutrophils; it increases the circulatory half-life of neutrophils from 8 to 48 hours.[47]

The Effects of GM-CSF on Neutrophil Function

GM-CSF has several effects on the function of neutrophils, including enhancement of neutrophil phagocytosis, antibody-dependent cellular cytotoxicity, chemotaxis, priming of the respiratory burst, and adhesion to endothelial cells.[47-51] Both GM-CSF and G-CSF inhibit programmed cell death or apoptosis of neutrophils, but the effects of GM-CSF on apoptosis are much more marked.[52]

The Mobilization of Hematopoietic Progenitors

In healthy adults, GM-CSF mobilizes fewer hematopoietic progenitors than G-CSF.[45,46] Lane and colleagues[45] compared the mobilization of hematopoietic progenitors in healthy donors who were given 10 μg/kg/day of GM-CSF for 4 days with donors who were given 10 μg/kg/day of G-CSF for the same amount of time. They found that, in the GM-CSF group, the mean CD34+ cell count increased to approximately 10×10^6 cells/L after 4 days compared with 60×10^6 cells/L in the G-CSF group. The number of BFU-E and CFU-GM that were mobilized in the GM-CSF group was also several-fold less than the number mobilized in the G-CSF group. In a similar study, Fritsch and colleagues[46] found that after 5 days of administering 5 μg/kg of G-CSF to healthy donors, their CD34+ cell count increased by a factor of 41.7 ± 27.2, but after 5 days of giving 5 μg/kg of GM-CSF to donors, the CD34+ cell count increased by a factor of 13.8 ± 4.9.

The Collection of Granulocytes and Peripheral Blood Progenitor Cells

The Collection of PBPCs

Circulating hematopoietic progenitor cells are collected with centrifugal blood cell separators through the use of procedures developed to collect mononuclear cells. The collections are usually started after G-CSF has been given to donors for 3-5 days.[1-7] Since peripheral venous access can be difficult to obtain on consecutive days, many centers attempt to collect enough cells for a transplant with a single apheresis procedure, usually on the fifth day of a course of G-CSF. The duration of the apheresis procedure is typically 3-5 hours in which 10-20 L of whole blood is processed.

The Composition of PBPCs

While the aim of PBPC collections is to harvest a variety of hematopoietic progenitor cells, the lack of generally-agreed-upon assays makes evaluation of their composition challenging. Most centers assess the quality of their concentrates through the use of flow cytometry to quantitate the number of CD34+ cells present. When 5-10 μg/kg/day of G-CSF was given for 5 days to 150 healthy donors and PBPCs were collected once, on the sixth day, the median number of CD34+ cells collected per liter of whole blood processed was 39.9×10^6 cells/L.[38] During the collection procedure, 8 or 9 L of whole blood was processed, and the median number of CD34+ cells collected was 330×10^6. Other studies have found that 41,[53] 34,[39] and 35×10^6 CD34+[54] cells can be collected per liter of whole blood processed.

Some investigators insist upon a functional assay of progenitor cells even though the results will not be available for several days to weeks. PBPCs also contain a large number of CFCs. In a study by Prosper et al,[43] healthy people were given 7.5 or 10 μg/kg of G-CSF for 5 days, and PBPCs were collected on the sixth day by processing 8-9 L of blood. The median number of CD34+ cells was 424 × 10^6, the median number of BFU-E was 34 × 10^6, the median number of CFU-GM was 66.7 × 10^6, and the median number of LTC-ICs was 5.1 × 10^6.[43]

Although PBPC collections are rich in hematopoietic cells, the most abundant cell is the platelet. The median number of platelets in 150 PBPC collections from donors who were given 5-10 μg/kg/day of G-CSF was 470,000/μL, and the range was 250,000-920,000/μL (Table 6-1).[38] This is similar to the quantity of platelets obtained in a plateletapheresis procedure, so if the PBPCs are transfused immediately after collection, then the transplant recipient also receives the effect of a platelet transfusion. On the other hand, some donors become significantly thrombocytopenic, and it is sometimes prudent to remove the platelets from the collection and return them to the donor. The large number of platelets in the PBPC collection may also make further processing of the unit difficult.

The PBPCs contained 11.9 to 163.9 × 10^9 of leukocytes. The most abundant leukocytes were lymphocytes and monocytes. The median percent of lymphocytes in the 150 PBPC collections was 67.5%, and the median percent of monocytes was 22.3% (Table 6-2).[38] The mean number of T lymphocytes (CD3+ cells) was 15.8 × 10^9, which is about 10 times the number in a marrow collection.[38] The median proportion of the leukocytes in the PBPCs that were neutrophils was 2.0%, and the range was 0-37% (Table 6-2). The median volume of red cells was 7.6 mL, and the range was 0-22 mL. In general, the red blood cell content of PBPCs does not exceed 1-1.5 mL of packed red blood cells per liter of whole blood processed.[54]

The Quantity of CD34+ Cells in PBPCs

Hematopoietic progenitors constitute a relatively small percentage of the cells in the PBPCs. In most cases, 4-5 × 10^6 CD34+ cells per kilogram weight of a recipient must be collected for an allogeneic transplant.[1] In a study by Stroncek et al,[38] 10 μg/kg/day of G-CSF was given to 67 healthy donors for 5 days, and cells were collected through the use of an apheresis procedure that processed 8-9 L of blood. The median number of CD34+ cells in the PBPCs was 383 × 10^6, enough to transplant a 76-kg person. However, the number of CD34+ cells that were collected varied from 78-1,380 × 10^6 and, for some donors, even two collections may not provide a sufficient number of cells for a transplant. In 10% of the donors, two 9-L collections provided only 4 × 10^6 CD34+ cells/kg or less for a 70-kg recipient, not enough for a transplant (Fig 6-3).[38]

The wide range in the number of CD34+ cells that can be collected from healthy donors is due in part to a variability in the number of CD34+ cells

Table 6-1. Effects of G-CSF Dose on the Quantity of Cells Collected From 150 Healthy Donors Who Were Given G-CSF for 5 Days Through One Apheresis Procedure

	Number of Cells Collected											
	5 μg/kg/day G-CSF (n = 25)			7.5 μg/kg/day G-CSF (n = 67)			10 μg/kg/day G-CSF (n = 58)			All Components (n = 150)		
Cell Type	**Mean ± SD**	**Median**	**Range**	**Mean ± SD**	**Median**	**Range**	**Mean ± SD**	**Median**	**Range**	**Mean ± SD**	**Median**	**Range**
WBCs ($\times 10^9$)	26.5 ± 9.0	25.4	11.9-56.2	34.0 ± 11.1	32.5	16.4-74.7	39.8 ± 21.8	36.0	15.6-163.3	35.0 ± 16.4	32.4	11.9-163.3
Mononuclear cells ($\times 10^9$)	25.9 ± 8.4	25.4	11.9-51.1	31.9 ± 8.6	31.4	14.9-58.5	38.1 ± 19.4	34.5	15.6-139.6	33.3 ± 14.4	31.4	11.9-139.6
CD34+ cells ($\times 10^6$)	276 ± 189	214.0	91-767	428 ± 300	336.0	70-1658	452 ± 294	383.0	78-1380	412 ± 287	330.0	70-1658
CD34+ cells ($\times 10^6$/L processed)	32.2 ± 21.2	24.8	9.9-90.0	51.5 ± 36.4	44.4	7.7-193.5	53.2 ± 33.1	46.5	9.3-146.3	48.4 ± 33.7	39.9	7.7-193.5
RBC (mL)	5.4 ± 4.7	6.3	0-19.0	8.0 ± 3.9	7.6	0-22.1	7.2 ± 3.5	7.6	0-15.5	7.2 ± 4.0	7.6	0-22.1
Neutrophils ($\times 10^9$)	0.64 ± 1.11	0.26	0-5.1	2.06 ± 4.3	0.69	0-27.6	1.77 ± 3.37	1.05	0-23.68	1.71 ± 3.59	0.64	0-27.6
Platelets ($\times 10^9$)	430 ± 80	420.0	300-630	490 ± 120	480.0	300-920	490 ± 100	490.0	250-740	480 ± 110	470.0	250-920

SD = standard deviation; WBCs = white blood cells; RBC = red blood cell.

(Used with permission from Stroncek et al.[38])

Table 6-2. Types of Leukocytes in 150 PBPC Collections From Healthy Donors Who Were Given 5, 7.5, or 10 μg/kg of G-CSF for 5 Days

Cell Type	Mean ± SD (%)	Median (%)	Range (%)
Lymphocytes	65.6 ± 13.7	67.5	27.0-93.0
Monocytes	22.5 ± 8.8	22.3	3.0-49.0
Neutrophils	3.6 ± 5.2	2.0	0-37
Bands	0 3 ± 0.9	0	0-8
Metamyelocytes	0.4 ± 1.0	0	0-5
Myelocytes	6.0 ± 5.8	5	0-39
Promyelocytes	0.5 ± 1.1	0	0-5
Blasts	0.4 ± 1.0	0	0-4
Basophils	0.7 ± 0.9	0.5	0-4

SD = standard deviation

The median volume of whole blood processed during the collection was 8.4 L.

(Used with permission from Stroncek et al.[38])

that are mobilized. The number of CD34+ cells that can be collected is related to WBC and neutrophil counts in the donor, but it is most closely related to the donor's precollection CD34+ cell count.[38] Because the number of CD34+ cells that are mobilized varies greatly among healthy donors, so does the number of CD34+ cells that can be collected.

Age is another factor that influences the number of CD34+ cells that can be collected. Anderlini and colleagues[55] found that the number of CD34+ cells collected per liter of blood processed was less in people over age 55 (25.2×10^6 CD34+ cells/L of blood processed) than in people less than or equal to 55 (35.6×10^6 CD34+ cells/L of blood processed). Another study[38] concluded that age does not influence the number of CD34+ cells collected; however, the subjects in that study were not old enough for researchers to see an effect that might not appear until after 55 years of age.

The number of CD34+ cells that can be collected is also correlated with the donor's weight and gender. Stroncek et al[38] noted that more CD34+

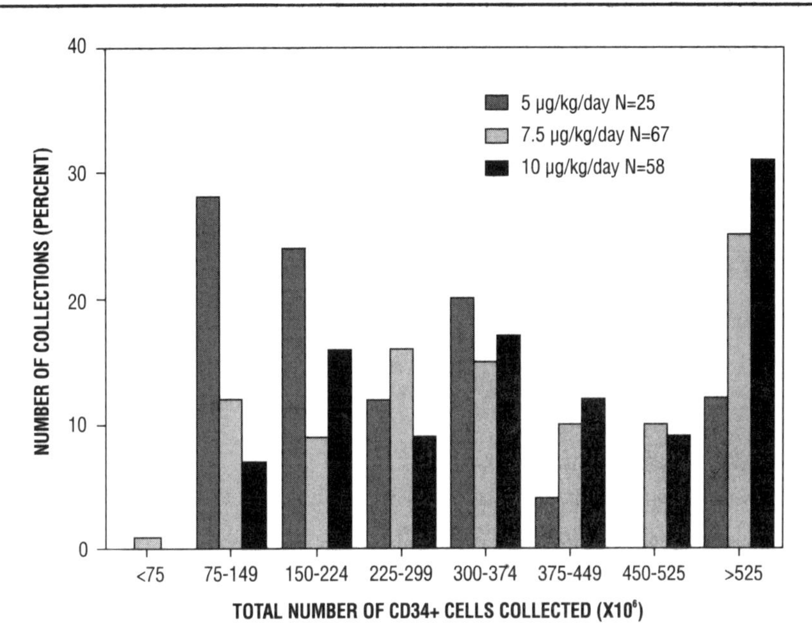

Figure 6-3. The effect of G-CSF doses on the quantity of CD34+ cells in 150 PBPC collections. Healthy donors were given 5, 7.5, or 10 µg/kg of G-CSF for 5 days and PBPCs were collected once, on the sixth day. The median volume of blood processed during the collection was 8.4 L. The PBPCs were grouped according to the quantity of CD34+ cells and the dose of G-CSF given. The number of PBPCs in each group was expressed as a percentage of all PBPCs that were collected from donors who were treated with each dose of G-CSF. (Used with permission from Stroncek et al.[38])

cells were collected from heavier people, and more were collected from males than from females. However, although donor gender and weight are related, it is not certain whether they exert independent effects on the number of cells that are collected.

The Number of PBPCs Required

While a single 9-L apheresis procedure may yield enough CD34+ cells for a transplantation, many healthy adults have tolerated longer procedures. Routine collections of 12-15 L were first used by sibling donors, but now as much as 20 L of whole blood is processed.[1-5] However, when the large-volume procedures are used, donors frequently experience symptoms resulting from citrate toxicity, and calcium must often be added to the blood return line. Even when 12-20 L of whole blood is processed during each collection procedure, two procedures must be performed to collect an adequate number of CD34+ cells in up to 33% of allogeneic transplant procedures.[56] In rare cases, three apheresis procedures must be performed.

Because of the great variability in the number of CD34+ cells in the PBPCs, the number of cells collected must be quantitated after each procedure. Unfortunately, the correlation between the precollection CD34+ cell counts and the number of CD34+ cells collected is not great enough to predict whether a single collection will be adequate for successful transplantation (Fig 6-4).[38] The number of CD34+ cells must be measured immediately after each collection; if the number is insufficient, then another collection must be performed.

Because the number of CD34+ cells in the circulation falls rapidly if the daily G-CSF injections are halted,[45] the injections must be continued as long as additional collections are anticipated. The optimal timing of the G-CSF injection on a day when PBPCs are collected remains uncertain. One study involving healthy donors who were given 2 μg/kg/day of G-CSF found that the number of circulating progenitor cells increased within 4-6 hours after a G-CSF injection.[28] Another study in which healthy donors were given 7.5-10 μg/kg/day of G-CSF found that there was no change in circulating CD34+ cell counts within 6 hours of an injection.[36] Giving the injection before the collection fits better into the routine of the apheresis center, but if the G-CSF makes the donor feel uncomfortable, then the collection could be more difficult.

Blood Cell Separators

Several types of blood cell separators can be used to collect PBPCs. The two instruments used most often are continuous flow centrifugation devices: the Fenwal CS3000 Plus (Baxter Biotech, Deerfield, IL) and the Spectra Apheresis System (COBE BCT Inc., Lakewood, CO). Discontinuous flow devices such as the V-50 or MCS blood cell separators (Haemonetics Corporation, Braintree, MA) can collect mononuclear cells, but they generally are not used because longer processing times are required. The discontinuous flow instruments have the advantage of allowing cells to be collected using single arm access. However, when venous access is problematic, femoral or central venous lines are usually preferred. During the collection procedure, whole blood is usually processed at a rate of 50-70 mL/minute, and citrate is used as an anticoagulant.

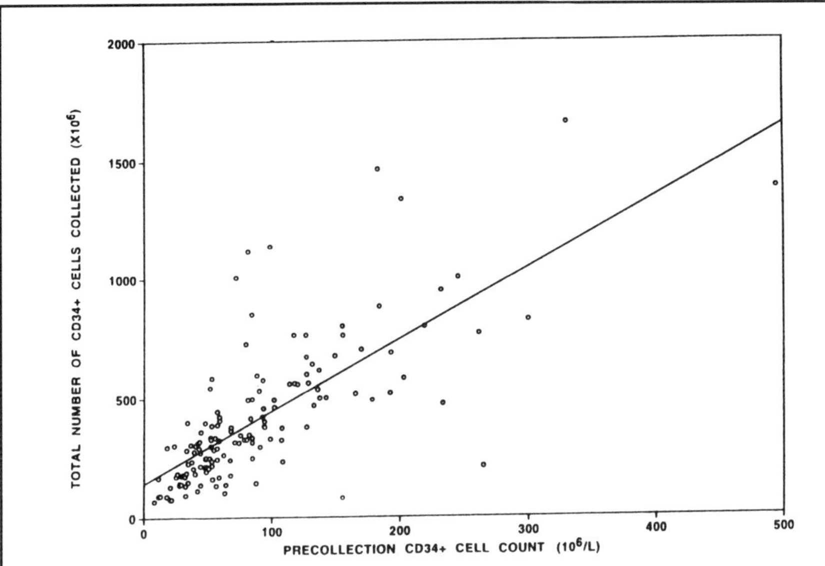

Figure 6-4. Correlation of the quantities of CD34+ cells in 150 PBPC collections from healthy donors with the blood CD34+ cell count before the collection. The donors were given 5, 7.5, or 10 µg/kg of G-CSF for 5 days and PBPCs were collected once, on the sixth day. Each point represents the total number of CD34+ cells in one PBPC collection and the CD34+ cell count in the donor's blood, which was measured on day 6 prior to the collection. The median volume of blood processed was 8.4 L. (Used with permission from Stroncek et al.[38])

Both of the continuous flow devices allow operator-initiated adjustments to optimize efficiency. With the CS3000 Plus, this includes adjustment of the interface detector setting from 100 to 140 as indicated by the precollection blood count and the use of a small-volume collection chamber to minimize platelet retention in the PBPCs. With the Spectra, the product collection rate can be altered from 0.8-1.5 mL/minute, and the hematocrit in the collection line can be adjusted for deeper or lighter penetration into the buffy coat layer.

The experience of two institutions using these two instruments is similar (Table 6-3).[54,57] Both blood cell separators are capable of collecting adequate numbers of CD34+ cells. A longer time interval is required for the establishment of a stable WBC layer in the Spectra and, as a result, the efficiency in collecting mononuclear cells using the Spectra is less than that of the CS3000 Plus. The PBPCs collected with the CS3000 Plus also contain fewer neutrophils.[57]

Venous Access

Both the CS3000 Plus and the Spectra require the use of two separate intravenous lines to collect PBPCs. Peripheral venous access cannot be obtained in 10-20% of the donors. If venous access for the PBPC collection cannot be obtained using peripheral veins, then a central venous line must be placed and used. As a last resort, marrow must be collected. Unfortunately, the placement of a central line may be the greatest risk that the PBPC donor encounters. Subclavian, internal jugular, and femoral lines can be used. Femoral lines are considered to be the safest to place, but when femoral catheters are used, the donor must remain in bed. The complication rate associated with the placement of a central line is estimated 1-2%.

While PBPCs can be cryopreserved, the hematopoietic cells for most allogeneic PBPC and marrow transplantations are transfused immediately after they are collected. The patient's irradiation and chemotherapy are given so that they are completed at the same time that the hematopoietic cells are transfused. Some centers collect and cryopreserve the PBPCs before giving transplant recipients their pretransplantation irradiation and chemotherapy,[2] which provides more flexibility in planning collections. When PBPCs are cryopreserved, then a second course of G-CSF can be given later, and additional PBPCs can be collected. This is especially helpful when venous access is a problem.

The Collection of Granulocytes

Traditionally, dexamethasone has been given to donors to increase the number of circulating granulocytes and, consequently, the number of granulocytes that can be collected with a blood cell separator.[58] While a single dose of dexamethasone (8 mg orally) can double the absolute granulocyte count in healthy donors, the administration of a single 5 μg/kg dose of G-CSF increases the granulocyte count four-fold. The combination of G-CSF plus dexamethasone increases the count five- to six-fold.[8,9,11] When donors are given only dexamethasone, $2.3 \pm 0.67 \times 10^{10}$ granulocytes can be collected,[58] but when a single dose of 3-5 μg/kg G-CSF is given 12-18 hours prior to the collection, $6.88 \pm 2.1 \times 10^9$ cells/L of blood processed or 44×10^9 total granulocytes can be collected.[9] Other investigators have found that when 5 μg/kg of G-CSF was given to donors, the mean number of granulocytes collected was 42×10^9 and 41×10^9 cells.[9,11] When 5 μg/kg G-CSF plus 8 mg of dexamethasone were given to healthy donors, the number of granulocytes collected per liter of blood processed increased to

Table 6-3. PBPC Collections From Healthy Donors Who Were Given G-CSF: Comparison of Yields Using Two Cell Separators

Parameter	Leitman et al[54]			Stroncek et al[57]		
	CS3000 (n = 19)	Spectra (n = 5)	p	CS3000 (n = 15)	Spectra (n = 14)	p
Volume processed (L)	4.9 ± 0.8	4.5 ± 1.9	0.23	8.9 ± 1.0	8.4 ± 1.0	0.71
MNCs collected ($\times 10^9$)	17.3 ± 5.9	13.9 ± 3.4	0.22	39.6 ± 21.9	26.9 ± 5.6	0.02
CD34+ cells collected ($\times 10^6$)	202 ± 128	137 ± 75	0.28	470 ± 353	419 ± 351	0.69
Neutrophils (%)	21 ± 7	28 ± 14	0.11	4 ± 5	13 ± 17	0.19
Neutrophils collected ($\times 10^9$)	NA	NA		1.4 ± 1.9	5.5 ± 8.7	0.01
Platelets collected ($\times 10^9$)	245 ± 67	222 ± 53	0.54	507 ± 98	531 ± 116	0.54
MNC collection efficiency (%)	79 ± 15	58 ± 14	0 01	82 ± 55	53 ± 14	0.04
CD34+ collection efficiency (%)	77 ± 27	54 ± 17	0.08	87 ± 61	53 ± 14	0.07
CD34+ cells/L~($\times 10^6$)	40.7	30.2	0.28	55.9 ± 42.0	45.9 ± 37.9	0.59

MNCs = mononuclear cells; NA = Data not available.

Table 6-4. Incidence (%) of Symptoms in Healthy Donors Donating G-CSF-Mobilized PBPCs

Symptom	Stroncek et al[18] 10 μg/kg/day (n = 27)	Leitman et al[53] 10 μg/kg/day (n = 24)	Anderlini et al[59] 12 μg/kg/day (n = 40)	Grigg et al[31] 10 μg/kg/day (n = 15)
Bone pain	96	100	82	87
Headache	48	38	70	33
Fatigue	22	31	20	47
Myalgia	4	29	0	27
Nausea	15	8	10	0

$12.4 \pm 0.71 \times 10^9$ cells/L, and the total number of granulocytes collected increased to $77.5 \pm 10.5 \times 10^9$ cells/L.[10]

Complications Associated With the Mobilization and Collection of PBPCs

Donor Symptoms

G-CSF

Healthy donors experience a wide variety of symptoms when they are given G-CSF for 5 days.[18,27,53,59] The exact incidence of these symptoms varies slightly from study to study, but the most frequently reported symptoms are bone pain, myalgias, headache, and fatigue (Table 6-4).[18,31,53,59] When 2.5-10 μg/kg/day of G-CSF was given for 5 days, 81% of the donors took acetaminophen or ibuprofen to treat their symptoms.[18] When the incidence of symptoms was compared in people given 2.5, 5, 7.5, or 10 μg/kg/day of G-CSF, bone pain and myalgias increased with the dose of G-CSF, as did the ingestion of analgesics. Gender also influenced the symptoms reported. Women were more likely to experience fatigue, nausea, and night sweats. Age has not been found to influence the incidence of symptoms.[18]

The G-CSF-related symptoms experienced by healthy PBPC donors are severe enough to cause 38% of the donors to limit their physical activities, but not sufficiently debilitating to prevent them from performing their usual work activities.[60] However, in 6-8% of the healthy people given G-CSF, the symptoms are so severe that the G-CSF dose must be reduced, and in 2-6 % of all people given G-CSF, the symptoms are so severe that the administration of G-CSF must be discontinued.[18] After the last dose of G-CSF is given, the severity of the symptoms decreases over 24-48 hours. However, 5% of the healthy donors given G-CSF report that they have not recovered completely until 2 weeks after the last injection.[58]

The incidence of symptoms in granulocyte concentrate donors who are given only one dose of G-CSF has not been studied as extensively, but granulocyte donors are likely to have fewer symptoms because they usually receive only a single low dose of G-CSF (5 μg/kg/day). When dexamethasone is used to mobilize granulocytes, the donors often experience insomnia, restlessness, and increased blood pressure. There is insufficient experience with a combination of these agents to know whether symptoms will be similar, exacerbated, or possibly mitigated.

GM-CSF

GM-CSF can cause a number of symptoms, including bone pain, myalgia, headache, fatigue, anorexia, skin rashes, edema, fever, and flushing. However, when a dose of 10 μg/kg/day of GM-CSF was given to healthy donors for 5 days, it was well tolerated.[45] Donors experienced myalgia and fatigue, but these side effects were partially or completely ameliorated by acetaminophen. In rare cases, GM-CSF can cause pleural and pericardial inflammation and effusions, and venous thrombosis can occur, especially at higher doses.[61,62]

Changes in Blood Chemistries

G-CSF affects several blood chemistries in healthy donors (Table 6-5).[18,59] The most marked changes occur in serum alkaline phosphatase and lactate dehydrogenase (LDH) levels, both of which increase two- to three-fold. Increases also occur in uric acid, alanine aminotransferase (ALT) and sodium, but bilirubin, potassium, and magnesium decrease. The magnitude of the changes in alkaline phosphatase increases with the dose of G-CSF, but the changes in LDH, ALT, bilirubin, sodium, and potassium are not affected by the G-CSF dose. These changes have not caused serious clinical problems, but one donor did develop gout after receiving G-CSF. Most centers do not routinely monitor blood chemistries in healthy people during the administration of G-CSF.

Blood chemistries have not been measured in granulocyte donors who have been given a single dose of G-CSF, but changes in alkaline phosphatase, LDH, and bilirubin occur after one dose of G-CSF; these changes will probably occur in granulocyte donors. Because the changes in potassium, sodium, and ALT do not occur until at least 3 doses of G-CSF have been given, these levels are not likely to change in granulocyte donors.

Postcollection Cytopenias

Thrombocytopenia

Healthy donors often experience transient thrombocytopenia following one or more PBPC donations.[20] The platelet counts decrease both as a result of the loss of platelets in the PBPCs and the suppression of platelet counts by G-CSF.[18,63] Immediately following the collection, the donor's platelet counts fall 30-35% because of the loss of platelets in the PBPCs (Fig 6-5).[20] Following the collection, the platelet counts remain decreased and unchanged for about 4 days. One week after the collection, the platelet counts increase but remain below precollection levels. Ten days after the

Table 6-5. Changes in Serum Chemistries in Healthy Donors Who Donated G-CSF-Mobilized PBPCs

Test	Reference	Number of Donors Tested	Pre G-CSF	Post G-CSF
Sodium (mmol/L)	Stroncek et al[18]	34	139 ± 2	142 ± 2
Potassium (mmol/L)	Stroncek et al[18]	34	4.0 ± 0.3	3.7 ± 0.4
	Anderlini et al[59]	43	4.2 ± 0.3	3.7 ± 0.4
Alkaline Phosphatase (U/L)	Stroncek et al[18]	34	73 ± 20	179 ± 43
	Anderlini et al[59]	43	90 ± 54	181 ± 96
Lactate Dehydrogenase (U/L)	Stroncek et al[18]	20	452 ± 49	1307 ± 363
	Anderlini et al[59]	43	415 ± 121	1089 ± 477
Alanine Aminotransferase (U/L)	Stroncek et al[18]	34	28 ± 9	38 ± 21
Bilirubin (mg/dL)	Stroncek et al[18]	34	0.7 ± 0.3	0.4 ± 0.2
Magnesium (mg/dL)	Anderlini et al[59]	43	1.9 ± 0.1	1.8 ± 0.2
Uric Acid (mmol/L)	Anderlini et al[59]	43	309 ± 71	386 ± 77

collection, the platelet counts return to precollection levels, and 2 weeks after the collection, the counts generally rise above precollection levels. The platelet counts remain elevated 3 weeks after the collection, but by 6 weeks after the collection, the counts return to pre-G-CSF levels.[63]

With only one PBPC collection from a healthy donor with a normal platelet count, the counts rarely fall to less than 100,000/µL. However, with two or more PBPC donation procedures, the median platelet count falls to 112,000/µL, and the counts range from 77,000-186,000/µL.[63]

While the thrombocytopenia is due primarily to the loss of platelets from PBPC donation, there does appear to be an element of suppression of platelet production and subsequent rebound caused by G-CSF. When platelets are collected by apheresis from healthy donors, the donors' platelet counts fall to a similar degree, but the platelet counts immediately begin to increase and return to precollection levels in about 4 days.[64] The fact that platelet counts fall in healthy donors when G-CSF is given for 5 or more days, even when no PBPCs are collected, suggests that the suppression of

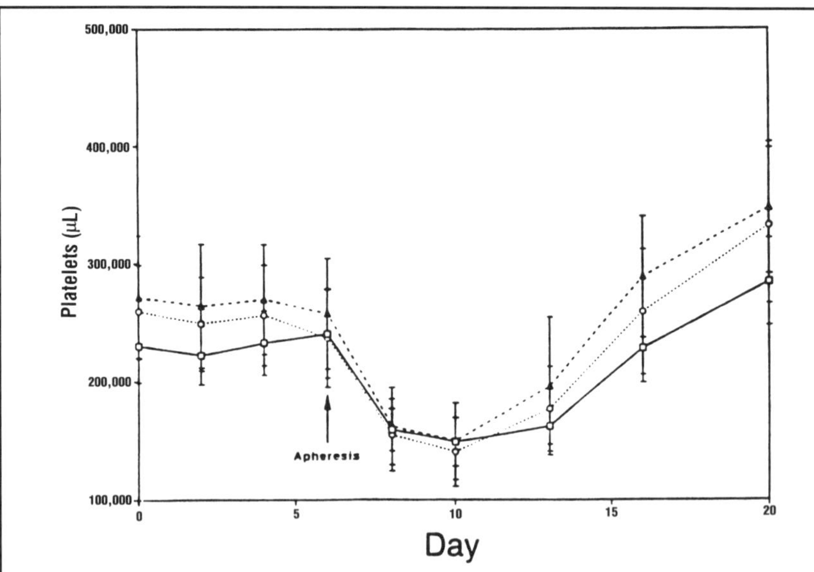

Figure 6-5. Thrombocytopenia following the collection of G-CSF-mobilized PBPCs. Platelet counts were measured in healthy donors who were given G-CSF for 5 days (days 1 - 5) and donated PBPCs once (day 6, arrow). The donors were given 5 (-□-, n = 9), 7.5 (-△-, n = 31), or 10 (-○-, n = 20) µg/kg per day of G-CSF. The values represent the mean ± SD. (Used with permission from Stroncek et al.[20])

platelet counts by G-CSF may be responsible for the delayed recovery of platelet counts in PBPC donors.[18] Evidence that G-CSF suppresses platelet counts for several days after the last dose has been given was provided by another study in which G-CSF was given to healthy donors for 5 days, but no PBPCs were collected.[63] In these people, the platelet counts fell below pre-G-CSF levels 4 days after the last dose was given and remained below pre-G-CSF levels 8 days after the last dose of G-CSF was given. The platelet counts rose above pre-G-CSF levels 2 weeks after the last dose was given.

Neutropenia

PBPC donors who have been given G-CSF experience a mild fall in neutrophil counts following the collection of PBPCs.[20,63,65] The neutrophil counts remain elevated for 4 days following the PBPC collection and then fall below the pre-G-CSF counts at 2 and 3 weeks following the collection.

The fall in neutrophil counts is mild. When 5-10 μg/kg/day of G-CSF was given for 5 days and PBPCs were collected, the mean absolute neutrophil count fell from 3.97×10^9 cells/L pre-G-CSF to 3.00×10^9/L 3 weeks after the collection.[20] Another study found that when 10 μg/kg of G-CSF was given for 5 days and PBPCs were collected twice, the median absolute neutrophil count fell from 3.3×10^9 cells /L (range = 2.3 to 5.8×10^9 cells /L) to 1.8×10^9 cells /L (range = 0.9 to 5.0×10^9 cells /L).[63] Postcollection infections have not been a problem, and this transient neutropenia does not appear to be of clinical significance.[20,65]

When G-CSF is given for 5 days but no PBPCs are collected, neutropenia does not occur.[62] This observation suggests that the neutropenia may be due to the loss of hematopoietic progenitor cells in the PBPCs.

Long-Term Follow-Up of Donors Given G-CSF

Only a limited number of donors of G-CSF-mobilized PBPCs have been evaluated one or more years later. No long-term ill effects on donors have been reported yet. Nineteen donors have had their blood counts measured 12-20 months after their donation. Hemoglobin, WBC count, WBC differential count, and platelet count were all normal (Table 6-6).[66] Blood counts and marrow biopsies performed in three people 5 years after they were given G-CSF were also normal.[67]

Results of the second collection of G-CSF-mobilized PBPCs several months after the first collection provide further evidence that G-CSF does not adversely affect the donor.[66,68] When a second course of G-CSF was given and more PBPCs were collected from 12 healthy people 12-20

Table 6-6. Comparison of Blood Counts in 19 Healthy Donors Who Were Measured Before Receiving G-CSF and 12-20 Months Later

	Counts Prior to G-CSF			Counts 1 Year Post G-CSF			
Cell Type	**Mean ± SD**	**Median**	**Range**	**Mean ± SD**	**Median**	**Range**	**p**
WBC (10^9/L)	5.94 ± 1.54	5.60	4.00-10.20	5.81 ± 1.57	5.40	4.00-10.10	0.69
Neutrophils (%)	62 ± 9	63.0	38-75	66 ± 10	69.0	47-82	0.13
Lymphocytes (%)	31 ± 10	30.0	17-57	27 ± 9	27.0	12-47	0.13
Monocytes (%)	5 ± 3	4.0	1-11	5 ± 3	4.0	0-10	0.74
Eosinophils (%)	2 ± 1	1.0	0-4	2 ± 2	2.0	0-8	0.39
Neutrophils (10^9/L)	3.68 ± 1.75	3.62	1.95-6.73	3.90 ± 1.46	3.62	2.08-7.58	0.68
RBC (10^{12}/L)	4.76 ± 0.45	4.70	4.00-5.43	4.72 ± 0.35	4.66	4.17-5.39	0.50
Hematocrit (%)	42 ± 4	43.0	36-47	42 ± 3	41.0	37-48	0.69
Platelets (10^9/L)	257 ± 51	254.0	169-352	274 ± 61	278.0	173-427	0.09
CD34+ (10^6/L)	6.45 ± 4.77	5.94	1.32-17.92	4.32 ± 2.23	4.21	1.62-9.36	0.10

SD = standard deviation; WBC = white blood cell; RBC = red blood cell.

(Used with permission from Stroncek et al.[66])

months following the first collection, the number of cells in each collection was very similar ($r_2 = 0.856$, $p<0.001$) (Fig 6-6).[66]

Children with congenital neutropenia have been given G-CSF regularly for up to 7 years.[69,70] Some of these children have developed leukemia or myelodysplasia, but it is not certain whether these hematologic abnormalities were part of the natural history of their disease, related to the administration of G-CSF, or due to a combination of the two factors.[69] No healthy donors who have been given a brief course of G-CSF have developed hematologic malignancies or marrow failure. However, it has been estimated that 2000 donors would have to be followed for 10 years to detect a 10-fold increase in the risk of developing leukemia due to G-CSF.[15]

The Use of Granulocyte Transfusions

Granulocyte transfusions can benefit patients who are neutropenic, infected with gram-negative bacteria, and are unresponsive to appropriate antibiotic therapy.[71] Infected patients who have inherited neutrophil func-

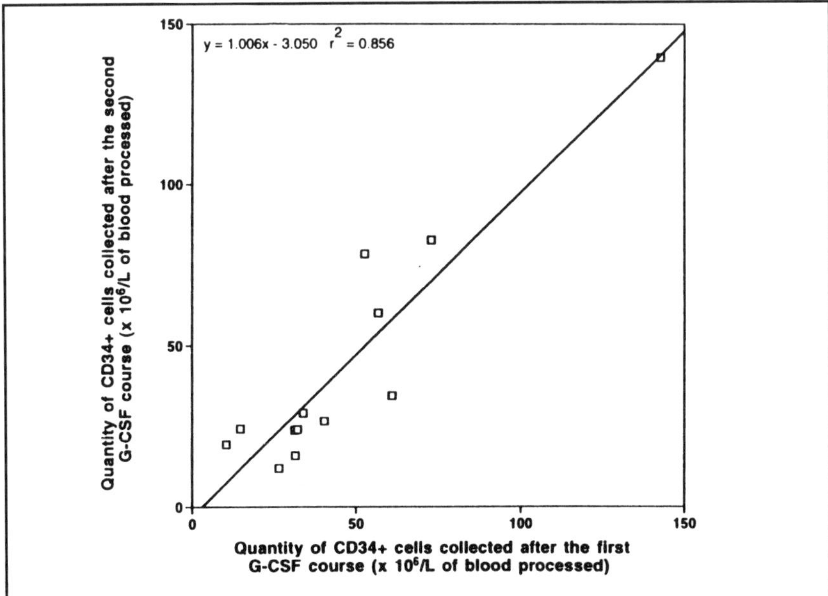

Figure 6-6. Comparison of the quantities of CD34+ cells collected per liter of blood processed through the use of two apheresis procedures in 12 healthy donors who were given 7.5 or 10 μg/kg of G-CSF during two courses of G-CSF, separated by 12.2 to 20.7 months. (Used with permission from Stroncek et al.[66])

tion defects, such as chronic granulomatous disease, also can benefit from granulocyte transfusions. Granulocyte transfusions have not proven to be effective in preventing infections in neutropenic patients or in treating fungal infections in neutropenic patients. However, the effectiveness of granulocyte transfusions in these situations may be limited by the quantity of cells that can be collected from the donors.

The transfusion of the 2×10^{10} granulocytes collected from donors who are stimulated with dexamethasone seldom results in a significant change of the granulocyte count of the transfusion recipient. Preliminary studies have found that the transfusion of the larger number of granulocytes, 4 to 8 $\times 10^{10}$, that can be collected from donors who are given G-CSF results in a significant increase in the granulocyte count of the transfusion recipient.[8-11] This increment is sustained for more than 24 hours, suggesting that in vivo survival is prolonged.[8-10] G-CSF-mobilized granulocytes have also been shown to exhibit delayed apoptosis in vivo, which may explain their prolonged circulating half-life. These results suggest that the granulocytes collected from donors treated with G-CSF or G-CSF plus dexamethasone may be more effective, but controlled studies investigating the effectiveness of G-CSF-mobilized granulocytes are needed. The availability of granulocyte concentrates containing several-fold increases in the number of cells and changes in the functional characteristics of the cells provide an opportunity to reevaluate and perhaps expand the therapeutic and prophylactic indications for granulocyte transfusions.

The Results of Transplants Using PBPCs

PBPCs are being used at many transplantation centers in place of marrow for allogeneic transplants involving HLA-compatible sibling donors. Several groups have retrospectively reported the results of patients who received allogeneic PBPC transplants for a variety of hematologic diseases (Table 6-7).

All the transplantation centers used G-CSF doses ranging from 5-16 μg/kg/day to mobilize the hematopoietic progenitors. The PBPCs were collected on days 5-7 of the G-CSF course. The G-CSF was given as a single morning dose or as a split morning and evening dose. The PBPCs were transfused immediately after collection, except at one center where the PBPCs were cryopreserved to ensure that a sufficient number of cells was collected.[2] The median dose of CD34+ cells transfused ranged from 4.2 to 13.1×10^6 CD34+ cells/kg of recipient weight, but as few as 1.8×10^6 cells/kg were given.

Table 6-7. Allogeneic G-CSF-Mobilized PBPC Transplants Using Sibling Donors

Investigator	Number of Patients	G-CSF dose (μg/kg) × days	Number of Collections (10 to 20 L each)	Median Number of CD34+ Cells Collected × 10^6/kg (range)	Median Number of CD3+ Cells Collected × 10^8/kg (range)	Median Days to		Acute GVHD	
						ANC >500/μL	Platelets >20,000/μL	Grade II, III, or IV	
Bensinger (95)[1]	8	16 × 5	2 (days 5,6)	13.1 (6.9-21.6)	3.85 (0.81-7.12)	14.5	10.5	2	1
Korbling (95)[2]	9	12 × 35	3 (days 4,5,6)	10.7 (7.5-22.5)	3.00 (1.27-15.23)	9*	12	3	0
Schmitz (95)[3]	8	5-10 × 5-6	1-3 (days 5,6,7)	6.7 (2.2-8.1)	3.40 (1 .95-4.18)	15.5	19.5	3	1
Azevedo (95)[5]	17	10 × 5	1 (day 6)	4.2 (1.8-13.8)	NA	14	14†	5	4
Majolino (96)[6]	9	10-16 × 4-5	1-2 (days 5,6)	6.8 (4.6-15.9)	2.07 (0.64-4.78)	13	15‡	2	0

ANC = absolute neutrophil count; GVHD = graft-vs-host disease; NA = data not available.

*All recipients were given G-CSF.

†>35,000 × 10^6 cells/L.

‡>50,000 × 10^6 cells/L.

Both neutrophil and platelet engraftment were rapid. The median time for the absolute neutrophil count to reach 500×10^6 cells/L ranged from 9-14.5 days, and the median time for the platelet counts to increase above 20,000/µL ranged from 10.5-19.5 days. One study compared the results of PBPC transplantation with allogeneic marrow transplantation performed at the authors' center during the same period and found that the time for neutrophil and platelet engraftment was faster in the patients who received PBPCs.[53] In addition, the PBPC transplant recipients had shorter hospital stays and used fewer antibiotics.

The median number of T cells (CD3+ cells) infused with the PBPCs ranged from 3.00 to 3.85×10^8 cells/kg, which is approximately 10 times the number in the typical marrow graft. Despite the large number of T cells given with the PBPCs, severe (Grade III or IV) graft-vs-host disease (GVHD) occurred in only six of 51 patients. Most of the patients were not followed long enough to assess the incidence of chronic GVHD, but one series found that patients who received PBPCs experienced a high incidence of chronic GVHD (75%) despite a low occurrence of acute GVHD (33%).[6]

Attempts have been made to reduce the incidence of GVHD by decreasing the number of T cells transplanted. Lymphocyte reduction is achieved generally by treating the PBPCs with a CD34+ cell immunoadsorption column. Although the number of T cells transplanted was reduced by 2 logs, eight of the 10 patients who were given the T-cell-reduced PBPCs developed severe (Grades III or IV) acute GVHD.[7]

One case-control study retrospectively compared the results of transplantation in patients with advanced hematologic malignancies using PBPCs from HLA-compatible siblings with transplant patients using marrow from HLA-compatible sibling donors.[4] Thirty-seven patients in each group were matched for age, gender, diagnosis, and disease phase. The results of this analysis were similar to those of the other reports. The time taken to reach a neutrophil count of 0.5×10^9 cells/L was less for recipients of PBPCs (14 days vs 16 days). The time taken to reach a platelet count of 20,000/µL independent of transfusions was also less in the recipients of the PBPCs (11 days vs 15 days). The PBPC recipient group also required fewer red blood cell transfusions (eight units compared with 17 units) and fewer platelet transfusions (24 units compared with 118 units).

There were no differences in the risk of acute or chronic GVHD in the two groups. The risk of developing acute GVHD (Grades II to IV) was 37% in the PBPC recipient group and 56% in the marrow recipient group. The risk of severe acute GVHD (Grades III to IV) was 14% in the PBPC group and 33% in the marrow group. Chronic GVHD occurred in seven of 18 evaluable PBPC recipients and in six of 23 evaluable marrow recipients.

Overall survival was also the same for both groups, 50% for the PBPC recipients and 41% for the marrow recipients.

Conclusions

G-CSF is being given routinely to allogeneic hematopoietic progenitor and granulocyte donors. The use of G-CSF-mobilized PBPCs for allogeneic transplantation is growing quickly. Initial studies of outcomes suggest that this procedure may replace marrow grafting for the majority of allogeneic transplantations involving HLA-compatible siblings. Granulocyte concentrates collected from donors who are given G-CSF may be more effective than those collected from donors who are treated with dexamethasone only, and the use of G-CSF-mobilized granulocytes will likely increase. Re-evaluation of the therapeutic and prophylactic use of granulocytes is indicated. The G-CSF treatments and apheresis collections induce several donor symptoms and changes in blood counts and chemistries. While these effects are generally well tolerated by healthy donors, much more study, especially of potential long-term effects, is important. G-CSF should be given only under the supervision of properly trained staff, and careful monitoring and follow-up are necessary. The collection of blood components from donors treated with G-CSF is an important new challenge for transfusion services and blood centers.

References

1. Bensinger WI, Weaver CH, Appelbaum FR, et al. Transplantation of allogeneic peripheral blood stem cells mobilized by recombinant human granulocyte colony-stimulating factor. Blood 1995;85:1655-8.
2. Korbling M, Przepiorka D, Huh YO, et al. Allogeneic blood stem cell transplantation for refractory leukemia and lymphoma: Potential advantage of blood over marrow allografts. Blood 1995;85:1659-65.
3. Schmitz N, Dreger P, Suttrop M, et al. Primary transplantation of allogeneic peripheral blood progenitor cells mobilized by filgrastim (granulocyte colony stimulating factor). Blood 1995;85:1666-72.
4. Bensinger WI, Clift R, Martin P, et al. Allogeneic peripheral blood stem cell transplantation in patients with advanced hematologic malignancies: A retrospective comparison with marrow transplantation. Blood 1996;88:2794-800.
5. Azevedo WM, Aranha FJP, Gouvea JV, et al. Allogeneic transplantation with blood stem cells mobilized by rh-G-CSF for hematological malignancies. Bone Marrow Transplant 1995;16:647-53.

6. Majolino I, Saglio G, Scime R, et al. High incidence of chronic GVHD after primary allogeneic peripheral blood stem cell transplantation in patients with hematologic malignancies. Bone Marrow Transplant 1996;17:555-60.
7. Link H, Arseniev L, Bahre O, et al. Transplantation of allogeneic CD34+ blood cells. Blood 1996;87:4903-9.
8. Bensinger WI, Price TH, Dale DC, et al. The effects of daily recombinant human granulocyte colony stimulating factor administration on normal granulocyte donors undergoing leukapheresis. Blood 1993; 81:1883-8.
9. Caspar CB, Seger RA, Burger J, Gmur J. Effective stimulation of donors for granulocyte transfusions with recombinant methionyl granulocyte colony-stimulating factor. Blood 1993;81:2866-71.
10. Leitman SF, Oblitas JM, Emmons R, et al. Clinical efficacy of daily G-CSF-recruited granulocyte transfusions on patients with severe neutropenia and life-threatening infections. Blood 1996;88:331a.
11. Hester JP, Dignani MC, Anaissie EJ, et al. Collection and transfusion of granulocyte concentrate from donors primed with granulocyte stimulating factor and response of myelosuppressed patients with established infection. J Clin Apheresis 1995;10:188-93.
12. Lieschke JM, Burgess AW. Granulocyte colony-stimulating factor and granulocyte-macrophage colony-stimulating factor. N Engl J Med 1992;327:28-35 Part 1, 99-106 Part 2.
13. Welte K, Gabrilove J, Bronchud MH, et al. Filgrastim (r-met Hu G-CSF): The first 10 years. Blood 1996;88:1907-29.
14. Demetri GD, Griffin J. Granulocyte colony-stimulating factor and its receptor. Blood 1991;78:2791-808.
15. Anderlini P, Przepiorka D, Champlin R, Korbling M. Biologic and clinical effects of granulocyte colony-stimulating factor in normal individuals. Blood 1996;88:2819-25.
16. Kwon EM, Sakamoto KM. The molecular mechanism of action of granulocyte-macrophage colony-stimulating factor. J Investig Med 1996;44:442-6.
17. Kerst JM, de Haas M, van der Schoot CE, et al. Recombinant granulocyte colony-stimulating factor administration to healthy volunteers: Induction of immunophenotypically and functionally altered neutrophils via an effect on myeloid progenitor cells. Blood 1993; 82:3265-72.
18. Stroncek DF, Clay ME, Petzoldt ML, et al. Treatment of normal individuals with G-CSF: Donor experiences and the effects on peripheral

blood CD34+ cell counts and the collection of peripheral blood stem cells. Transfusion 1996;36:601-10.

19. Chatta GS, Price TH, Allen RC, Dale DC. Effects of in vivo recombinant methionyl human granulocyte colony-stimulating factor on the peripheral blood colony-forming cells in healthy young and elderly adult volunteers. Blood 1994;84:2923-9.
20. Stroncek DF, Clay ME, Smith J, et al. Changes in blood counts following the administration of G-CSF and the collection of peripheral blood stem cells from healthy donors. Transfusion 1996;36:596-600.
21. Lord LI, Bronchud MH, Owens S, et al. The kinetics of human granulopoiesis following treatment with granulocyte colony-stimulating factor in vivo. Proc Natl Acad Sci USA 1989;86:9499-503.
22. Avalors BR, Gasson JC, Hedvat C, et al. Human granulocyte colony-stimulating factor: Biologic activities and receptor characterization on hematopoietic cells and small cell lung cancer cell lines. Blood 1990;75:851-7.
23. Kitagawa S, Yuo A, Souza LM, et al. Recombinant human granulocyte colony stimulating factor enhances superoxide release in human granulocytes stimulated by chemotactic peptide. Biochem Biophys Res Commun 1987;144:1143-7.
24. Yong KL, Linch DC. Differential effects of granulocyte and granulocyte-macrophage colony-stimulating factors (G- and GM-CSF) on neutrophil adhesion in vitro and in vivo. Eur J Haematol 1992;49: 251-9.
25. de Haas M, Kleijer M, van Zwieten R, et al. Neutrophil FcγRIIIb deficiency, nature and clinical consequences: A study of 21 individuals from 14 families. Blood 1995;86:2403-13.
26. Jutila MA, Rott L, Berg LE, Butcher EC. Function and regulation of the neutrophil Mel-14 antigen in vivo: Comparison with LFA-1 and Mac-1. J Immunol 1989;143:3318-24.
27. McCullough J, Clay ME, Hurd D, et al. Effect of leukocyte antibodies and HLA matching on the intravascular recovery, survival, and tissue localization of 111-indium labeled granulocytes. Blood 1986;67:522-8.
28. Matsunaga T, Sakamaki S, Kohgo Y, et al. Recombinant human granulocyte colony stimulating factor can mobilize sufficient amounts of peripheral blood stem cells in healthy volunteers for allogeneic transplantation. Bone Marrow Transplant 1993;11:103-8.
29. Dreger P, Haferlach T, Eckstein V, et al. G-CSF mobilized peripheral blood progenitor cells for allogeneic transplantation: Safety, kinetics of

mobilization and composition of the graft. Br J Haematol 1994; 87:609-13.

30. Fujisaki T, Otsaka T, Harada M, et al. Granulocyte colony-stimulating factor mobilizes primitive hematopoietic stem cells in normal individuals. Bone Marrow Transplant 1994;16:57-62.
31. Grigg AP, Roberts AW, Raumon H, et al. Optimizing dose and scheduling of filgrastim (granulocyte colony-stimulating factor) for mobilization and collection of peripheral blood progenitor cells in normal volunteers. Blood 1995;86:4437-45.
32. Harada M, Nagafuji K, Fujisaki T, et al. G-CSF induced mobilization of peripheral blood stem cells from healthy adults for allogeneic transplantation. J Hematother 1996;5:63-71.
33. Tjonnefjord GE, Steen R, Evensen SA, et al. Characterization of CD34+ peripheral blood cells from healthy adults mobilized by recombinant human granulocyte colony-stimulating factor. Blood 1994;84:2796-801.
34. Sate N, Sawada KI, Takahashi TA, et al. A time course study for optimal harvest of peripheral blood progenitor cells by granulocyte colony stimulating factor in healthy volunteers. Exp Hematol 1994;22:973-8.
35. Sica S, Rutella S, Di Mario A, et al. rhG-CSF in healthy donors: Mobilization of peripheral hematopoietic progenitors and effect on peripheral blood leukocytes. J Hematother 1996;5:391-7.
36. Stroncek DF, Clay ME, Herr G, et al. The kinetics of G-CSF mobilization of CD34+ cells in healthy individuals. Transfus Med 1997;7:19-24.
37. Walker CF, Bertz H, Wenger S, et al. Mobilization of peripheral blood progenitor cells for allogeneic transplantation: Efficacy and toxicity of a high-dose rhG-CSF regime. Bone Marrow Transplant 1996;18:279-83.
38. Stroncek DF, Clay ME, Smith J, et al. Composition of peripheral blood stem cell components collected from healthy donors. Transfusion 1997;37:411-7.
39. Korbling M, Huh YO, Durett A, et al. Allogeneic blood stem cell transplantation: Peripheralization and yield of donor-derived primitive hematopoietic progenitor cells (CD34+ thy-1dim) and lymphoid subsets, and possible predictors of engraftment and graft versus host disease. Blood 1995;86:2842-8.
40. Bender JG, Unverzagt K, Walker DE, et al. Phenotypic analysis and characterization of CD34+ cells from normal human bone marrow, cord blood, peripheral blood, and mobilized peripheral blood from pa-

tients undergoing autologous stem cell transplantation. Clin Immunol Immunopathol 1994;70:10-8.

41. Steen R, Tjonnefjord GE, Egeland T. Comparison of the phenotype and clonogenicity of normal CD34+ cells from umbilical cord blood, granulocyte colony-stimulating factor-mobilized peripheral blood and adult human bone marrow. J Hematother 1994;3:253-62.
42. Prosper F, Stroncek D, Verfaillie CM. Homing of mobilized PBPC, which adhere poorly to stroma due to low levels of VLA-4, may result from upregulation of expression and function of VLA-4 once PBPCs are removed from the mobilized milieu (abstract). Blood 1996; 88(Suppl):475a.
43. Prosper F, Stroncek D, Verfaillie CM. Mobilization of long-term culture initiating cell (LTC-IC) in normal donors treated with G-CSF: Phenotypic analysis and characterization of primitive progenitors in mobilized PBSC. Blood 1996;88:2033-42.
44. Papayannopoulou T, Nakamoto B. Peripheralization of hematopoietic progenitors in primates treated with anti-VLA4 integrin. Proc Natl Acad Sci USA 1993;90:9374-8.
45. Lane T, Law P, Maruyama M, et al. Harvesting and enrichment of hematopoietic progenitor cells mobilized into the peripheral blood of normal donors by granulocyte-macrophage colony stimulating factor (GM-CSF) or G-CSF: Potential role in allogeneic marrow transplantation. Blood 1995;85:275-82.
46. Fritsch G, Fishmeister G, Haas OA, et al. Peripheral blood hematopoietic progenitor cells of cytokine-stimulated healthy donors as an alternative for allogeneic transplantation. Blood 1994;83:3420-1.
47. Vadas MA, Nicola NA, Metcalf D. Activation of antibody-dependent cell-mediated cytotoxicity of human neutrophils and eosinophils by separate colony-stimulating factors. J Immunol 1983;130:795-801.
48. Fleishmann J, Golde DW, Weisbart RH, Gasson JC. Granulocyte-macrophage colony-stimulating factor enhances phagocytosis of bacteria by human neutrophils. Blood 1986;68:708-11.
49. Weisbart RH, Kwan L, Golde DW, Gasson JC. Human GM-CSF primes neutrophils for enhanced oxidative metabolism in response to the major physiological chemoattractants. Blood 1987;69:18-25.
50. Wang JM, Chen ZG, Colella S, et al. Chemotactic activity of recombinant human granulocyte colony stimulating factor. Blood 1988;72: 1456-60.
51. Arnaout MA, Wang EA, Clark SC, Sieff CA. Human recombinant granulocyte-macrophage colony-stimulating factor increases cell-to-

cell adhesion and surface expression of adhesion-promoting glycoproteins on mature granulocytes. J Clin Invest 1986;78:597-602.
52. Brach MA, de Vos S, Gruss H-J, Herrmann F. Prolongation of survival of human polymorphonuclear neutrophils by granulocyte-macrophage colony stimulating factor is caused by inhibition of programmed cell death. Blood 1992;80:2920-4.
53. Leitman SF, Sekhsaria S, Gladden D, et al. Safety and efficacy of recombinant granulocyte colony-stimulating factor (G-CSF) in mobilizing blood stem cells in healthy donors (abstract). Transfusion 1995;35 (suppl):66S.
54. Leitman SF, Read EJ. Hematopoietic progenitor cells. Semin Hematol 1996;33:341-58.
55. Anderlini P, Przepiorka D, Seong D, et al. Factors affecting mobilization of CD34+ cells in normal donors treated with filgrastim. Transfusion 1997;37:507-12.
56. Anderlini P, Przepiorka D, Huh Y, et al. Duration of filgrastim mobilization and apheresis yield of CD34+ progenitor cells and lymphoid subsets in normal donors for allogeneic transplantation. Br J Haematol 1996;93:940-2.
57. Stroncek DF, Clay ME, Smith J, et al. Comparison of two blood cell separators in collecting peripheral blood stem cell components. Transfus Med 1997;7:95-9.
58. Lee J-H, Leitman SF, Klein HG. A controlled comparison of the efficacy of hetastarch and pentastarch in granulocyte collections by centrifugal leukapheresis. Blood 1995;86:4662-6.
59. Anderlini P, Przepiorka D, Seong D, et al. Clinical toxicity, laboratory effects, and analysis of charges for filgrastim mobilization and blood stem cell apheresis from normal donors. Transfusion 1996;36:590-5.
60. Stroncek DF, Clay ME, Lennon S, et al. Collection of two stem cell components from healthy donors (abstract). Transfusion 1996;36 (suppl):26S.
63. Stephens LC, Haire WD, Schmidt-Porkny K, et al. Granulocyte macrophage colony stimulating factor: High incidence of apheresis catheter thrombosis during peripheral stem cell collection. Bone Marrow Transplant 1993;11:51-4.
62. Socinski MA, Cannistra SA, Elias A, et al. Granulocyte-macrophage colony stimulating factor expands the circulating haematopoietic progenitor cell compartment in man. Lancet 1988;1:1194-8.
63. Stroncek D, Clay M, Lennon S, et al. Neutropenia following the collection of granulocyte-colony stimulating factor mobilized blood pro-

genitor cell components is due to the collection of progenitor cells (abstract). Blood 1996;88:396a.

64. Lasky LC, Lin A, Kahn RA, McCullough J. Donor platelet response and production quality assurance in plateletpheresis. Transfusion 1981; 21:247-60.
65. Anderlini P, Przepiorka D, Seong D, et al. Transient neutropenia in normal donors after G-CSF mobilization and stem cell apheresis. Br J Haematol 1996;94:155-8.
66. Stroncek DF, Clay ME, Herr G, et al. Blood counts in healthy donors 1 year after the collection of granulocyte-colony-stimulating factor-mobilized progenitor cells and the results of a second mobilization and collection. Transfusion 1997;37:304-8.
67. Sakamaki S, Matsunaga T, Hirayama Y, et al. Haematological study of healthy volunteers 5 years after G-CSF. Lancet 1995;346:1432-3.
68. Anderlini P, Laupee J, Przepiorka D, et al. Peripheral blood stem cell apheresis in normal donors: Feasibility and yield of second collections. Br J Haematol 1997;96:415-7.
69. Dale DC. Hematopoietic growth factors for the treatment of severe chronic neutropenia. Stem Cells 1995;13:94-100.
70. Bonilla MA, Dale M, Zeidler C, et al. Long-term safety of treatment with recombinant human granulocyte colony-stimulating factor (r-metHu-G-CSF) in patients with severe congenital neutropenias. Br J Haematol 1994;88:723-30.
71. Strauss RG. Therapeutic granulocyte transfusions in 1993. Blood 1993;81:1675-8.

In: Davenport RD, Snyder EL, eds.
Cytokines in Transfusion Medicine: A Primer
Bethesda, MD: AABB Press, 1997

7

Thrombopoietic Agents

RAZA A. KHAN, MD, AND JOHN W. SMITH II, MD

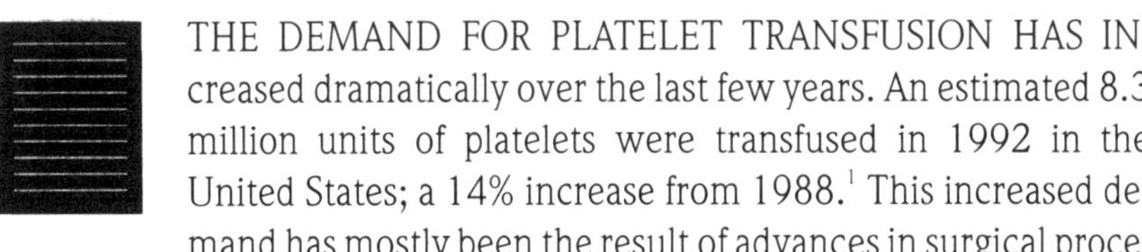

THE DEMAND FOR PLATELET TRANSFUSION HAS INcreased dramatically over the last few years. An estimated 8.3 million units of platelets were transfused in 1992 in the United States; a 14% increase from 1988.[1] This increased demand has mostly been the result of advances in surgical procedures such as cardiac surgery, organ transplants, including bone marrow transplants, and the use of dose-intensive chemotherapy for cancer patients. These procedures often promote thrombocytopenia in recipients, thus creating a need for platelets. Thrombocytopenia also results from peripheral platelet destruction, as in trauma, infection, or immune thrombocytopenic purpura. Bleeding may result from quantitative and qualitative disorders of platelet function resulting from intrinsic errors occurring within the megakaryocyte.

Raza A. Khan, MD, Fellow, Hematology/Oncology, Department of Internal Medicine, University of Michigan, Ann Arbor, Michigan; and John W. Smith II, MD, Chief, Clinical Research, Earle A. Charles Research Institute, Providence Portland Medical Center, Portland, Oregon

Approximately 3.6 million platelet units transfused in 1992 were collected through single-donor apheresis procedures in order to limit alloimmunization and transmission of infection to the recipient from the donor. This adds considerable cost and time to meet the increasing demand for platelet transfusions.

An understanding of the biochemical and molecular mechanisms underlying thrombopoiesis rests on an understanding of the development of the platelet within its precursor cell, the megakaryocyte, as the platelet lacks a nucleus. The study of megakaryocytes has been difficult because of the low numbers and fragility of these cells. Megakaryocytes respond to thrombopoietic demand in a highly regulated and complex process in which several regulatory signals work in concert on the megakaryocytic microenvironment consisting of cells, growth factors, and extracellular matrix to achieve this response. Marrow is the major site of platelet production; extramedullary sites include the spleen and lungs, which account for 7-15% of the production process.[2]

The cellular components of the megakaryocytic microenvironment within the marrow include the parenchymal cells committed to the megakaryocyte lineage and the neighboring stromal cells such as fibroblasts, endothelial cells, and macrophages. These stromal cells produce growth factors and extracellular molecules that are needed for megakaryocyte function.

Megakaryocyte Lineage

Megakaryocytes arise from the most primitive multi- or pluripotential hematopoietic stem cells that are capable of giving rise to cells of different lineages. Committed progenitor cells arise from these cells through a defined series of cellular stages.

Megakaryoblasts

The earliest cells of the megakaryocytic line are defined functionally. The first detectable cell in this lineage is the megakaryocyte high-proliferative-potential colony-forming cell (Mk-HPP-CFC). The burst-forming unit–megakaryocyte (BFU-Mk) is more mature than the Mk-HPP-CFC. The most differentiated proliferating cell is the colony-forming unit–megakaryocyte (CFU-Mk). The BFU-Mk are CD34+ HLA-DR–, while the more mature CFU-Mk are CD34+ HLA-DR+.

Promegakaryoblasts

Promegakaryoblasts (PMkBs) are transitional cells intermediate between the megakaryoblast and the mature megakaryocytes. Three antigenically distinct subpopulations of human PMkB can be identified on the basis of the coexpression of CD34 and platelet glycoprotein IIIa (GPIIIa) (GPIIIa, CD41). CD34+ GPIIIa– are the most primitive, CD34+ GPIIIa+ are intermediate, and CD34– GPIIIa+ are the most mature of these cells.

Megakaryocytes

Megakaryocytes (Mks) are the first cells in the megakaryocyte lineage that can be morphologically recognized. Mature megakaryocytes rarely express CD34. They variably express platelet factor 4, platelet glycoprotein IIb/IIIa, von Willebrand factor (vWF), thrombospondin, and thrombomodulin.

Platelets

The final event in the megakaryocyte lineage is the release of platelets into the circulation. Proliferation and invagination of the megakaryocyte plasma membrane occurs, resulting in the demarcation membrane system (DMS) that divides the megakaryocyte cytoplasm into platelet fields. Finally, the megakaryocyte seems to extend pseudopods into the sinusoidal lumen from which platelets are shed into the circulation. Platelets are small anuclear cells containing α granules and dense bodies (δ granules) in the cytoplasm. The α granule contains adhesive proteins, growth modulators, and coagulation factors, the dense body contains agonists like adenosine diphosphate (ADP), adenosine triphosphate (ATP), serotonin, and calcium, as well as the cytokines RANTES and macrophage inflammatory protein-1α (MIP-1α).[3] Platelet surface receptors and their ligands, including GPIa/IIa—collagen, GPIb/IX—vWF, GPIc/IIa—fibronectin, and VLA-6—laminin, are involved in platelet adhesion. GPIIb/IIIa interacts with fibrinogen in the early phase of aggregation.

The Effects of Cytokines on Platelet Production

Although the existence of a lineage-specific regulator of platelet production was speculated for a long time, the study of megakaryocyte development both in vivo and in vitro was hampered by the scarcity of megakaryocytes in the marrow, poorly defined cell populations, and inadequate assays. It was postulated that this regulator of platelet production would increase the number of megakaryocytes, as well as increase the size, ploidy, and the rate of maturation of these megakaryocytes in order to increase the number of platelets in response to thrombocytopenia. Two types of factors were hypothesized to accomplish this process: 1) early acting megakaryocyte colony-stimulating factors (MEG-CSFs) and 2) late-acting megakaryocyte maturation factors called thrombopoietins (TPOs).[4] This model was similar to the other blood cells that are controlled by the early- and late-acting factors; for example, c-*kit* ligand (c-*kit*) and erythropoietin (EPO) for erythropoiesis, granulocyte macrophase colony-stimulating factor (GM-CSF) and macrophage colony-stimulating factor (M-CSF) for monocytes, interleukin-3 (IL-3) and interleukin-5 (IL-5) for eosinophils, and IL-3, GM-CSF, or c-*kit* and granulocyte colony-stimulating factor (G-CSF) for neutrophils.

The quest for MEG-CSF and thrombopoietin led to a series of experiments to isolate these factors from serum, plasma, and urine of thrombocytopenic humans and animals as well as conditioned cultured media from various cell lines. Efforts were also made to test various cytokines for their ability to limit chemotherapy-induced thrombocytopenia. This resulted in a number of laboratory and clinical studies of GM-CSF, interleukin-1 (IL-1), IL-3, IL-3 agonists, the artificial agonist PIXY321, interleukin-6 (IL-6) and interleukin-11 (IL-11), leukemia inhibitory factor (LIF), and most recently TPO.

Granulocyte Macrophage Colony-Stimulating Factor

GM-CSF stimulates development of the multilineage progenitor cell CFU-granulocyte-erythroid-macrophage megakaryocyte (GEMM) as well as BFU-Mk and CFU-Mk. However, the activity of GM-CSF in stimulating platelet production in vivo is relatively weak compared with its actions on leukocyte precursors. Cell culture experiments demonstrate that its megakaryocyte-stimulatory activity is approximately 1/100th of that of IL-3. GM-CSF functions as a megakaryocyte CSF, and its actions are additive to those of IL-3.[5] The additive nature of these two cytokines is also seen in PIXY321, a genetically engineered fusion protein containing the functional domains of IL-3 and GM-CSF.

Both GM-CSF and G-CSF have been used to decrease the severity and duration of neutropenia and the number of days of febrile neutropenia in chemotherapy-treated cancer patients. These clinical trials have not consistently demonstrated an increase in platelet count. In one study, patients who were treated with high-dose chemotherapy and radiation followed by autologous bone marrow transplant were randomly assigned to receive GM-CSF. The patients who received GM-CSF required fewer platelet transfusions and had a higher platelet nadir.[6] Other studies have not confirmed these results.[7]

Although G-CSF has no direct platelet-augmenting activity, it can increase the number of circulating CD34+ stem cells and has been used for priming patients for peripheral blood progenitor cell (PBPC) harvest through the use of apheresis. G-CSF-primed PBPC transplantation has been demonstrated to shorten the duration of thrombocytopenia and decrease requirements for platelet transfusion in patients receiving high-dose chemotherapy.[8]

Interleukin-1

Interleukin-1 has a variety of activities such as direct antitumor cytotoxicity, enhancement of the resistance to bacterial sepsis, and protection against the myelosuppressive effects of radiation and chemotherapy. IL-1 induces the production of many cytokines including IL-6 and G-CSF. In addition, IL-1 upregulates the expression of receptors for IL-1, G-CSF, and IL-3 on hematopoietic progenitor cells. These activities are reviewed in the first chapter of this book.

Phase I trials of IL-1 in cancer patients resulted in significant toxicity, including hypotension that required presser support.[9] Other toxicities included fever, chills, nausea, vomiting, fatigue, headache, abdominal pain, edema, confusion, and prerenal azotemia. A dose-dependent increase in neutrophils and total leukocytes and a significant increase in platelets above pretherapy baseline were noted. In one such trial, interleukin-1 alpha (IL-1α) was given to patients before and after receiving high-dose carboplatin. When given after chemotherapy, platelet recovery time to 100,000/μL was significantly reduced.[10] In another trial in which IL-1 was given to ovarian cancer patients, significantly less thrombocytopenia was seen in patients who received the cycle containing carboplatin followed by IL-1 than in patients who received the preceding cycle with carboplatin alone.[11] Despite promising evidence of enhanced platelet recovery, IL-1 is currently not being used in clinical trials because of its toxicity profile.[9]

Interleukin-3

Interleukin-3 is capable of inducing the proliferation and differentiation of multipotent hematopoietic stem cells and the growth of committed erythroid, megakaryocyte, granulocyte and macrophage progenitors in vitro. It stimulates immature as well as mature megakaryocytes.[12] Exogenous IL-3 stimulates the in vivo expansion of megakaryocyte progenitor cells, but by itself, IL-3 has a limited effect on platelet production.[13] In vivo, IL-3 is only produced by antigen-activated T lymphocytes, which suggests that its role in maintaining basal hematopoiesis or platelet production is minimal.

In Phase I trials, IL-3-induced flu-like symptoms (fever, chills, and headaches).[13] Modest increases in the platelet nadir following chemotherapy were observed in the Phase II trials. The use of IL-3 after autologous bone marrow transplantation has been less promising. A large Phase III study compared IL-3 with placebo in patients with relapsed and progressive primary lymphoma who were being treated with ifosfamide, epirubicine, and etoposide.[14] There was no difference in the need for platelet transfusions in the two groups. Another study compared the use of IL-3 followed by GM-CSF with GM-CSF alone in patients with Hodgkin's and non-Hodgkin's lymphoma.[5] There was no difference in the number of platelet transfusions or infectious complications in these two groups.

The results of these trials suggest that IL-3, when used alone or in combination with GM-CSF, has only modest effects on platelet counts, platelet nadirs, and platelet recovery. However, because IL-3 acts earlier in megakaryocytopoiesis than TPO, it may be beneficial to administer both in combination or sequence.

IL-3 Receptor Agonists

IL-3 receptor agonists are synthetic cytokines produced from a library of protein ligands of the human IL-3 receptor. Synthokine (SC-55494) was produced to enhance the growth-promoting activities of IL-3 without increasing its histamine and leukotriene releasing properties.[15,16] Synthokine stimulates CFU-G, -M, -GM, -GEMM, and -Mk, and BFU-E. It is also a potent stimulator of mature and progenitor cell expansion ex vivo alone and in synergy with IL-6, G-CSF, GM-CSF, and c-*kit*. Synthokine studies in irradiated rhesus monkeys showed a decrease in the number of days when platelet levels were less than 20,000/μL.[17]

PIXY321 is a fusion protein composed of GM-CSF that is connected to IL-3 by a flexible linker protein. This compound binds to a 100-kD cell surface receptor that is distinct from the IL-3 or GM-CSF receptors.[18] A Phase I/II clinical trial that was conducted with PIXY321 showed granulocyte-augmenting effects similar to GM-CSF and an inconsistent increase in platelet recovery after chemotherapy.[19] Recently, results of a Phase III trial of PIXY321 has failed to show a benefit for thrombocytopenia.[20] PIXY321 was shown to be no different than GM-CSF after chemotherapy for breast cancer, lymphoma, and after bone marrow transplantation.[19,20] Moreover, the company sponsoring trials of PIXY321 has stopped clinical development of this agent.

Interleukin-6

Interleukin-6 performs has biologic activities. It affects human megakaryocytopoiesis, stimulates B cells, differentiates cytotoxic T cells, and stimulates the synthesis of acute-phase reactants by the liver. IL-6 stimulates megakaryocyte maturation and its actions are partially additive to those of IL-3.[2,4] A consensus of studies indicates that IL-6 is elevated in patients with reactive, but not primary, thrombocytosis.[21-23] Furthermore, there have been no observations of a reciprocal correlation relationship between IL-6 levels and platelet count.

In Phase I trials of IL-6, flu-like symptoms, nephrotoxicity, neurotoxicity, and cardiotoxicity were observed in a dose-related fashion.[24-26] Preliminary results from a Phase II trial showed only modest effects in patients with sarcoma or lung cancer who are treated with chemotherapy.[27] Because of its toxicity/efficacy profile, development of IL-6 has been stopped by its manufacturers.

Interleukin-11

Interleukin-11 is encoded by a gene located on chromosome 19. It was initially cloned from a primate marrow stromal cell line. IL-11 has multiple effects on in vitro and in vivo megakaryocytopoiesis, affecting both early hematopoietic stem cells and progenitor cells as well as enhancing megakaryocyte maturation that results in an increased ploidy of megakaryocytes. IL-11, along with IL-1 and c-*kit* ligand, interacts with IL-3 at the level of BFU-Mk. IL-11 synergizes with IL-3 to shorten the G_0 period of early hematopoietic progenitors. IL-6 and IL-11 seem to use the same signal transduction pathway, although they bind to different receptors.

A Phase I trial involving 16 patients with Stage III-B and IV breast cancer who were receiving cyclophosphamide and doxorubicin and 10-100 μg/kg/day of IL-11 demonstrated tolerance at doses below 50 μg/kg/day.[28] Grade II constitutional symptoms and extremity edema were seen in all patients at 75 μg/kg/day. Fevers were not observed in any patients. At 100 μg/kg/day, one patient developed transient expressive aphasia. Another patient with history of hypertension developed cerebral infarct. A transient anemia, not dose-related, was seen in all patients. Further evaluation suggested the anemia was a result of volume expansion. Elevation of acute-phase proteins was seen at all levels. A 76-180% dose-related increase in platelet counts was seen above baseline at various dose levels. No change in platelet aggregometry was seen with IL-11 therapy. Marrow biopsies demonstrated a significant increase in the number of megakaryocytes at doses of 50 μg/kg/day or more. No effects on the number of committed progenitors were noted. Flow cytometric analysis showed an increase in ploidy of megakaryocytes, demonstrating the effects on cell maturation. IL-11 had no significant effect on neutrophil counts, and patients were safely given G-CSF for neutropenia while on IL-11.

In a Phase I/II trial, the toxicity and efficacy of rh (recombinant human) IL-11 were studied. rhIL-II was administered to patients after they received ifosfamide, carboplatin, and etoposide (ICE) chemotherapy. Eleven patients were treated with ICE followed by G-CSF (5 μg/kg/day) and IL-11 (25, 50, and 75 μg/kg/day) until the absolute neutrophil count and platelet count recovered to 1,000,000/μL and 100,000/μL, respectively. There were no episodes of Grade III/IV toxicity to rhIL-11. All 11 patients had Grade IV hematologic toxicity. The median time for the recovery of the platelet count to 100,000/μL was 21 days (25 μg/kg/day), 18.5 days (50 μg/kg/day), and 22 days (75 μg/kg/day). The median number of platelet transfusions following chemotherapy, IL-11, and G-CSF was two. Compared with a previous trial, conducted by the same authors, in which patients received ICE and G-CSF alone, preliminary data suggest that IL-11 (50 μg/kg/day) and G-CSF after ICE might decrease the total number of platelet transfusions (12 vs 2) and accelerate platelet recovery (27 vs 19 days).[29]

Tepler et al[30] recently conducted a multicenter, randomized, placebo-controlled trial of rhIL-11 involving 93 cancer patients who had already been transfused platelets for severe thrombocytopenia resulting from chemotherapy. The patients had received platelet transfusion for a nadir platelet count of less than 20,000/μL during the chemotherapy cycle that immediately preceded the study entry. Chemotherapy was continued during the study without dose reduction. Patients were randomly selected to receive placebo or rhIL-11 at 25 or 50 μg/kg subcutaneously once daily for 14-21 days beginning one day after chemotherapy. Eight (30%) of 27 patients treated with rhIL-11 at a dose of 50 μg/kg did not require platelet transfusions compared with one (4%) of 28 patients who received placebo ($p<0.05$). Five (18%) of 27 patients treated with rhIL-11 at 25 μg/kg avoided platelet transfusions (p = NS vs placebo). Side effects were fatigue and cardiovascular symptoms, including a low incidence of atrial arrhythmia and syncope. There were no differences among treatment groups in the incidence of neutropenic fever, days of hospitalization, or number of red blood cell transfusions. This study shows that IL-11 treatment at a dose of 50 μg/kg/day significantly increases the likelihood that patients who have already received platelet transfusions for chemotherapy-induced thrombocytopenia will not require platelet transfusions during a subsequent chemotherapy cycle.

Thrombopoietin

Cloning and Expression

None of the agents described above seemed to fulfill the requirements of the postulated thrombopoietin. The successful cloning of thrombopoietin began when an important discovery was made in an unrelated field when the myeloproliferative leukemia virus (MPLV) was identified. In 1986, Wendling et al[31] described a transforming viral complex that induced a myeloproliferative syndrome in the recipient mice. Four years later, the transforming gene v-*mpl* was identified in 1990,[32] and, in 1992, the cellular homologue of viral gene, proto-oncogene c-*mpl*, was identified and was found to be specifically involved in megakaryocyte regulation.[33]

The search for the ligand of c-*mpl* led to the isolation and cloning of thrombopoietin, which was reported independently by three different groups in 1994.[34-36] Groups at Genentech (San Francisco, CA) and Amgen (Thousand Oaks, CA) used affinity chromatography using c-*mpl* receptors. Groups at the University of Washington (Seattle, WA) and ZymoGenetics (Seattle, WA) used chemical mutagenesis to generate a cell line that produced murine TPO; specific cDNA was then obtained by functional expression cloning technique. Later, two more groups, Ogami et al and Kuter et al, independently reported the isolation of TPO using protein fractionation methods from thrombocytopenic rats and rabbits respectively.[37,38] Subsequent results suggested that c-*mpl* ligand, thrombopoietin, and CSF-Mk might be the same molecule.[39] The ligand for c-*mpl* was found to be relatively lineage-specific, working both alone and synergistically with early-acting cytokines to support megakaryocyte colony formation, and acting at a late stage of development to increase megakaryocyte size, polyploidization, and expression of markers.

In vivo, c-*mpl* ligand stimulates platelet production by greatly expanding marrow and splenic megakaryocytes and their progenitors and by shifting the distribution of megakaryocyte ploidy to higher values. Since the c-*mpl* ligand had the expected characteristics of the major regulator of megakaryocyte development, it was proposed that it be termed thrombopoietin.[40] TPO, c-*mpl* ligand, and megakaryocyte growth and development factor (MGDF) are all names for the same molecule.

One of the groups (ZymoGenetics) reported the functional cloning of a murine-complementary DNA that encodes a ligand for the receptor encoded by the c-*mpl* proto-oncogene.[36] The encoded polypeptide has a molecular mass of 35,000 Daltons. The protein has a novel two-domain structure with an amino-terminal domain homologous with erythropoietin and a carboxy-terminal domain rich in serine, threonine, and proline residues that contain seven potential N-linked glycosylation sites.[41,42] The gene for c-*mpl* ligand was found to be made up of seven exons and six introns spanning eight kilobases. The protein is encoded by exons 3-7. The human MGDF gene has been mapped to chromosome 3q26-27.[43-45]

TPO has a domain similar to human erythropoietin that encompasses the N-terminal half of the molecule. The C-terminal tail carries the majority of the glycosylation sites. The whole molecule has problems with stability; therefore, this molecule was truncated, retaining the EPO-like domain and splicing the glycosylated terminal. This truncated molecule was then conjugated to polyethylene glycol (PEG) to stabilize the molecule while retaining its biologic activity; it was termed MGDF or rhPEG-MGDF.

Thrombopoietin has been shown by Northern blot and reverse transcriptase-polymerase chain reaction (RT-PCR) analysis to be produced primarily in the liver and kidneys as well as in the spleen and marrow. Such a wide range of tissue types suggested that a common cell type, such as endothelium or fibroblasts, contributes to TPO production. RT-PCR of human and murine primary cells and cell lines reveals TPO-specific mRNA in endothelial and fibroblast-derived cells as well as hepatoma cell lines.[46]

The identification and cloning of the megakaryocyte-specific, c-*mpl* TPO have opened the door for rapid advances in our understanding of the processes of platelet regulation. TPO induces intracellular tyrosine phosphorylation. Events induced by TPO have been compared with the events stimulated by IL-3. The overall pattern of tyrosine phosphorylation stimulated by TPO and IL-3 in myeloid precursor cells revealed an overlapping but not identical pattern that reflects their distinct but partially redundant biologic effects.[47,48]

Hematopoietic Effects

The development of megakaryocytes from their marrow precursors is one of the least understood aspects of hematopoiesis. Current models suggest that early-acting, Mk colony-stimulating factors, such as IL-3 or c-*kit* ligand, are required for the expansion of hematopoietic progenitors into cells capable of responding to late-acting Mk potentiators, including IL-6 and IL-11. Thrombopoietin has been shown to display both Mk colony-stimulating factor and potentiator activities. Neutralizing the biologic activity of TPO eliminates Mk formation in response to c-*kit*, IL-6, and IL-11, alone and in combination, but only a partial reduction in Mk formation in the presence of combinations of cytokines including IL-3, although full maturation was not seen. Data indicate that two populations of Mk progenitors can be identified: one that is responsive to IL-3 but can develop fully only in the presence of TPO, and a second that is dependent on TPO for both proliferation and differentiation.[43]

Further studies have investigated the effects of various cytokines in combination with TPO. TPO activity is additive with IL-3 and synergistic with c-*kit* in causing an increase in CFU-Mk and platelets. Compared with IL-3, TPO action on human megakaryocytic cell lines enhances polyploidization up to 64N and surface membrane expression of GPIb and IIb/IIIa.[49-52]

To determine whether the activity of TPO was a result of other cytokines or stromal cell interactions, neutralization studies were performed. These studies used antisera to IL-3, GM-CSF, IL-1β, and IL-11. No diminution in TPO activity was observed in the presence of these antisera. The effects of TPO on interactions between human megakaryocytes and bone marrow stromal fibroblasts were studied. No changes were observed in either megakaryocyte expression of the surface molecules' lymphocyte function-associated antigen-1 (LFA-1), very late activation antigen-4 (VLA-4), intercellular adhesion molecule-1 (ICAM-1), or the adhesion of megakaryocytes to stromal fibroblasts after treatment with the growth factor. Furthermore, no induction of secretion or other cytokines, such as IL-1 α, IL-1 β, GM-CSF, IL-6, G-CSF, tumor necrosis factor-α, transforming growth factor-β1, or transforming growth factor-β2, by human megakaryocytes was noted after treatment of the cells with TPO.[53] TPO greatly expanded the number of erythroid progenitors and blood reticulocytes and was associated with accelerated red cell recovery in myelosuppressed mice.[54]

In addition to increasing the circulating platelet mass, TPO may have effects on platelet function. When TPO was added to normal human blood in concentrations of 10-100 ng/mL, a dose-dependent increase in both spontaneous and ADP-stimulated platelet activation was observed in an in-vitro experiment. A similar increase was also seen when TPO was administered to normal mice at doses sufficient to elevate the platelet count, resulting in a marked enhancement of both spontaneous platelet activation and ADP-induced platelet activation.[55] Thrombopoietin has been shown to enhance platelet aggregation induced by 2 mmol/L of ADP in a dose-dependent fashion. This enhancement is not affected by the treatment of platelets with aspirin and a thromboxane antagonist but is inhibited by a soluble form of the thrombopoietin receptor. Thrombopoietin (10 μg/mL) also enhances or primes platelet aggregation induced by collagen (0.5 mmL), thrombin, serotonin, and vasopressin.[56]

Animal studies were conducted to elucidate the regulation and relationship between low platelet counts and TPO.[57] To determine the relationship between blood levels of thrombopoietin and changes in the circulating platelet mass, rabbits were given subcutaneous busulfan. As the platelet mass declined, levels of thrombopoietin increased inversely and proportionally and peaked during the platelet nadir. When the platelet mass returned to normal, thrombopoietin levels decreased accordingly. When platelets were transfused into thrombocytopenic rabbits near the time of their platelet count nadir, the elevated levels of thrombopoietin decreased.

TPO levels in normal donors and in patients with abnormal platelet levels due to thrombocytopenia or thrombocytosis have revealed an inverse relationship with the platelet counts.[58] Plasma samples from normal donors (platelet counts between 100,000/µL and 500,000/µL) had a mean TPO level of 85 ± 6.7(SEM), thrombocytopenic patients (platelet counts less than 100,000/µL) had a mean TPO level of 4571 ± 2135 pg/mL, and thrombocytic patients (platelet counts greater than 500,000/µL) had a mean TPO level of 339 ± 101 pg/mL.

In another study,[59] TPO levels were measured in aplastic anemia patients and idiopathic thrombocytopenic purpura (ITP) patients using enzyme-linked immunosorbent assay (ELISA). TPO levels were undetectable in 60 normal volunteers using this assay. Eight aplastic anemia patients who ultimately responded to immunosuppressive therapy had low platelet counts (mean 23,000/µL, range 5000-61,000/µL), and all had markedly elevated TPO levels (mean 1517 pg/mL, range 710-2880). TPO levels measured after platelet counts recovered (mean 134,000/µL, range 92,000-175,000/µL) were substantially decreased (mean 440 pg/mL, range 193-771). In marked contrast, TPO levels were all below the limit of detection in 18 patients with chronic ITP and severe thrombocytopenia (mean 19,000/µL, range 1000-60,000/µL). This study raised the possibility that TPO production is constant and that the major determinant of TPO levels may be the megakaryocyte mass that binds TPO from the circulation and degrades it, rather than the platelet number. The authors proposed that TPO levels may help differentiate thrombocytopenia resulting from peripheral destruction (such as ITP) where megakaryocyte mass is high from thrombocytopenia resulting from marrow failure (such as aplastic anemia) where megakaryocyte mass is low.

Additional support of this concept is provided by the studies generating "knock-out" mice, in which the animals missing the gene for the TPO receptor (c-*mpl*) were created, resulting in an 85% decrease in blood platelet count.[60] It was noted that normal platelets bind and internalize TPO, while "knock-out" platelets did not bind TPOs at all, demonstrating the role of TPO receptors in this regulation.

Another proposal is that c-*mpl* expression is a regulated event influenced by the feedback provided by the megakaryocytes or platelets.[61] In order to identify the molecular basis for this regulation, TPO mRNA levels from selected organs of mice with high, normal, or low platelet counts were subjected to semiquantitative RT-PCR. These data suggest that TPO levels are regulated, at least in part, by modulating mRNA levels in response to platelet demand.

The effects of rHuMGDF on megakaryocytopoiesis in normal nonhuman primates have been studied.[62] rHuMGDF was administered subcutaneously to normal, male rhesus monkeys once per day for 10 consecutive days at dosages of 2.5, 25, or 250 μg/kg of body weight. Circulating platelet counts increased significantly ($p<0.05$) for all doses within 6 days of rHuMGDF administration and reached maximal levels between 12 and 14 days after cytokine administration. The 2.5, 25.0, and 250.0 micrograms/kg/day doses elicited peak mean platelet counts that were 592%, 670%, and 449% of baseline, respectively. Marrow-derived, clonogenic data showed significant increases in the concentration of CFU-Mk and CFU-GEMM, whereas that of GM-CFU and burst-forming unit-erythroid (BFU-E) remained unchanged during the administration of rHuMGDF.

Clinical Trials

Data from the first, randomized, double-blind, placebo-controlled Phase I trial of PEG-rHuMGDF have been presented in abstract form.[63] PEG-rHuMGDF was given to patients before (cycle 0) and after (cycle 1) receiving dose-intensive chemotherapy in order to determine the safety and minimum clinically effective dose of PEG-rHuMGDF. The patients were treated with PEG-rHuMGDF, or with placebo, at planned PEG-rHuMGDF dose levels of 0.03, 0.1, 0.3, 1.0, 3.0, and 5.0 μg/kg/day subcutaneously for 10 days, followed by at least 3 washout days. Chemotherapy was given 1 day later followed by blinded study drug at the dose given in cycle 0 plus G-CSF 5 μg/kg, subcutaneously until hemopoietic recovery or for 21 days, whichever was earlier. The first abstract reported on 11 patients (seven males, four females), median age 61 years (range 36-74), with a variety of advanced solid tumors. Eleven patients completed cycle 0 and eight completed cycle 1. In cycle 0, four of 11 patients demonstrated a 95-395% increase in platelet counts over baseline values, peaking at 12-16 days after the start of the blinded study drug administration. No toxicity attributable to MGDF had been observed. In the most recent update, a total of 31 patients were treated with MGDF and 10 with placebo in the second phase of this study where MGDF was given after chemotherapy.[64] The drug was initially given for 20 days; however, the last three cohorts received the drug for 10 days only. Nadir counts were the same in the two groups but platelet counts returned to normal earlier in the MGDF group, analogous to G-CSF. Recovery to baseline platelet count was 18 days for the MGDF group vs 26 days for the placebo group ($p<0.15$). Moderate increases in platelet counts were seen at 0.03 and 0.1 μg/kg. Increases in platelet counts at 0.3 and 1.0 μg/kg occurred by day 7. Peak platelet counts of 800,000/μL, 1,300,000/μL, and 1,800,000/μL were noted at a 1.0 μg/kg dose between day 14 and 17. No effects on absolute granulocyte count or RBC parameters were seen. No fever, inflammation, weight gain, or increase in fibrinogen were noted.

Marrow histopathology was assessed at baseline and at day 8. Blinded histopathologic assessment of marrow revealed both qualitative and quantitative changes in megakaryocytes. Despite peak platelet counts of up to 942,000/μL, no significant alteration in platelet surface markers, aggregation, or ATP release has been detected. These preliminary data suggest no evidence of in vivo platelet activation or hyperaggregation.[65]

The latest update also reported the effects on progenitor cells in marrow and peripheral blood. There was no change in the level of progenitor cells in marrow. However, bone marrow megakaryocytes were increased at all dose levels, including a two-fold increase at 1.0 μg/kg. Progenitor cells of all lineages were mobilized into peripheral blood. There was a median three-fold increase and a maximum 30-fold increase in megakaryocyte progenitors. The increase in granulocyte and macrophage progenitors was similar to G-CSF in magnitude, but persisted longer.

Another Phase I placebo-controlled trial of PEG-rHuMGDF was conducted in patients with lung cancer who were receiving carboplatin and paclitaxel.[66] In Cycle 0, PEG-rHuMGDF was given for 10 days before chemotherapy. In Cycle 1, PEG-rHuMGDF was given for up to 17 days after chemotherapy. G-CSF was not given in this trial. PEG-rHuMGDF doses were 0.1, 0.03, 1.0, 3.0, and 5.0 μg/kg/day subcutaneously. A total of 53 patients received the study drug before and/or after chemotherapy. Fifty patients received the study drug in the postchemotherapy phase, 38 received MGDF, and 12 received placebo. The median platelet nadir after chemotherapy was 189,000/μL with MGDF compared to 111,000/μL with placebo ($p = 0.019$). Recovery to baseline platelet count was 14 days with MGDF vs more than 21 days with the placebo ($p<0.001$). Administration of MGDF for as few as 3 days was found to be effective. Toxicity observed in some patients included deep venous thrombosis and pulmonary embolism in one patient who had a platelet count of 250,000/µL and was treated with MGDF at 3 µg/kg for 7 days. Superficial thrombophlebitis was seen in one patient who had a platelet count of 780, 000/µL and was treated with MGDF at 1 µg/kg. A Grade II drug rash was observed in one patient. No effects on weight, blood pressure, or serum chemistries were seen. There were no detectable antibodies to MGDF.

Results of a study using a single dose of rhTPO have been reported in abstract form.[67] In the first cycle, TPO was given to patients as a single dose 21 days before chemotherapy and, in the second cycle, TPO was given to patients as a single dose after chemotherapy. TPO doses ranged from 0.3-2.4 µg/kg (three patients per group in each study). A total of 18 patients were treated. A 60-200% increase in platelets above baseline was observed. Peak platelet counts were seen on day 12 but platelet counts were still significantly higher than baseline on day 21. Megakaryocytes were increased up to four-fold in the marrow. The platelets appeared normal in morphology and exhibited a normal response to aggregation in response to various agonists. No change occurred in either white blood cells or RBCs. Mild transient headaches developed in six out of 18 patients. One patient developed nonneutralizing antibodies.

Conclusions

It is apparent that a number of pharmaceutic products are now, or shortly will be, available that significantly influence platelet production. Preliminary results of clinical trials clearly suggest that several of these agents are effective in increasing platelet counts and reducing the need for platelet transfusions in the settings of chemotherapy-induced myelosuppression and marrow transplantation. However, indications for the use of hematopoietic growth factors to stimulate platelet production have yet to be completely defined. In the next few years, it is likely that one or two factors, such as TPO and IL-11, could markedly decrease, but certainly not eliminate, the need for platelet transfusions.

References

1. Wallace EL, Churchill WH, Surgenor DM, et al. Collection and transfusion of blood and blood components in the United States, 1992. Transfusion 1995;35:802-12.
2. Smith EB, Butcher J. The incidence, distribution and significance of megakaryocytes in normal and diseased human tissues. Blood 1952; 7:214-24.

3. Klinger MHF, Wilhelm D, Bubel S, et al. Immunocytochemical localization of chemokines RANTES and MIP-1α within human platelets and their release during storage. Int Arch Allergy Immunol 1995;107: 541-6.
4. Gewirtz AM, Schick B. Megakaryocytopoiesis. In: Colman RW, Hirsch J, Marder VJ, Salzman EW, eds. Hemostasis and thrombosis: Basic principles of clinical practice. 3rd ed. Philadelphia: JB Lippincott, 1994:353-96.
5. Fay JW, Felser JM, Abboud C, et al. Sequential administration of recombinant human interleukin-3 (IL-3) and granulocyte-macrophage colony-stimulating factor (GM-CSF) after autologous bone marrow transplantation (ABMT) therapy for lymphoma: Results of a phase III multi-center study (abstract). Blood 1995;86:222a.
6. Brandt SJ, Peters WP, Atwater SK, et al. Effects of recombinant granulocyte macrophage colony stimulating factor on hematopoietic reconstitution after high dose chemotherapy and autologous bone marrow transplantation. N Engl J Med 1988;318:869-76.
7. Nemunaitis J, Rabinowe SN, Singer JW, et al. Recombinant granulocyte macrophage colony stimulating factor after autologous bone marrow transplantation for lymphoid cancer. N Engl J Med 1991;324: 1773-8.
8. Chao NJ, Schriber JR, Grimes K, et al. Granulocyte colony stimulating factor "mobilized" peripheral blood progenitor cells accelerate granulocyte and platelet recovery after high dose chemotherapy. Blood 1993;81:2031-6.
9. Salvatore V, Smith JW II. Interleukin I trials in cancer patients: A review of toxicity, antitumor and hematopoietic effects. Stem Cells 1996;14:164-76.
10. Smith JW II, Longo DL, Alvord WG, et al. The effects of treatment with interleukin 1α on platelet recovery after high-dose carboplatin. N Engl J Med 1993;328:756-61.
11. Vadhan-Raj S, Kudeka A, Garrison L, et al. Effects of interleukin 1α on carboplatin-induced thrombocytopenia in patients with recurrent ovarian cancer. J Clin Oncol 1994;12:707-14.
12. Kavnoudias H, Jackson H, Ettlinger K, et al. Interleukin 3 directly stimulates both megakaryocyte progenitor cells and immature megakaryocytes. Exp Hematol 1992;20:43-6.
13. Ganser A, Lindemann A, Seipelt G, et al. Effects of recombinant human interleukin-3 in patients with normal hematopoiesis and in pa-

tients with bone marrow failure. Phase I/II study. Blood 1990;76: 666-76.

14. Gerhartz HH, Mandelli F, Philip T, et al. Randomized phase III study of interleukin-3 (rhIL-3) in IEV-chemotherapy of relapsing aggressive lymphomas (abstract). Blood 1995;86:54a.
15. McKearn JP, Bauer C, Klein B, et al. Evaluation of a synthetic cytokine of human IL-3 receptor with significantly improved activity relative to native IL-3 (abstract). Blood 1994;84:422a.
16. Hood WF, Thomas JW, Kahn LE, et al. Binding analysis of a synthetic cytokine to high and low affinity of the IL-3 receptors (abstract). Blood 1994;84:421a.
17. Farese AM, Herodin F, Grab LB, et al. Therapeutic efficacy of Synthokine SC-55494 in a nonhuman primate model of high dose sublethal, radiation-induced hypoplasia (abstract). Blood 1994;84:28a.
18. Bruno E, Briddell RA, Cooper RJ, et al. Recombinant GM-CSF/IL-3 fusion protein: Its effect on in vitro human megakaryocytopoiesis. Exp Hematol 1992;20:494-9.
19. O'Shaughnessy JA, Tolcher A, Riseberg D, et al. Prospective, randomized trial of 5-Fluorouricil, Leucovorin, Doxorubicin and Cyclophosphamide chemotherapy in combination with the interleukin-3/granulocyte-macrophage colony-stimulating factor (GM-CSF) fusion protein (PIXY321) versus GM-CSF in patients with advanced breast cancer. Blood 1996; 87:2205-11.
20. Vose JM, Pandite L, Beveridge RA, et al. Phase III study comparing PIXY321 and GM-CSF following autologous bone marrow transplantation (ABMT) in patients with non-Hodgkin's lymphoma (NHL) (abstract). Blood 1995;86:972a.
21. Hollen CW, Henthorn J, Koziol JA, Burstein SA. Elevated serum interleukin-6 levels in patients with reactive thrombocytosis. Br J Haematol 1991;79:286-90.
22. Gangarossa S, Romano V, Munda SE, et al. Low serum levels of interleukin-6 in children with post-infective acute thrombocytopenic purpura. Eur J Haematol 1995;55:117-20.
23. Kuyama J, Take H, Matsumoto S, et al. Synchronous fluctuation of interleukin-6 and platelet count in cyclic thrombocytopenia and thrombocytosis. Intern Med 1995;34:636-9.
24. Weber J, Yang JC, Topalian SL, et al. Phase I trial of subcutaneous interleukin-6 in patients with advanced malignancies. J Clin Oncol 1993;11:499-506.

25. Weber J, Gunn H, Yang J, et al. A phase I trial of intravenous interleukin-6 in patients with advanced cancer. J Immunother 1994; 15:292-302.
26. Van Gameren MM, Willemse PHB, Mulder NH, et al. Effects of recombinant human interleukin-6 in cancer patients: A phase I-II study. Blood 1994;84:1434-41.
27. Budd GT, Pelley R, Samuels B, et al. Phase II randomized trial of simultaneous rhIL-6 and G-CSF following MAID chemotherapy in patients with sarcomas: Preliminary results (abstract). Proc Annu Meet Am Soc Clin Oncol 1995;14:694.
28. Gordon MS, McCaskill-Stevens WJ, Battiato LA, et al. A phase I trial of recombinant human interleukin-11 (Neumega rhIL-11 growth factor) in women with breast cancer receiving chemotherapy. Blood 1996;87:3615-24.
29. Ali-Nazir A, Davenport V, Reaman G, et al. Preliminary results of a phase I/II study of rhIL-11 following ifosfamide, carboplatin, and etoposide (ICE) chemotherapy in pediatric patients (pts) with solid tumors (st) or lymphoma (l): enhancement of hematological reconstitution (abstract). Blood 1995;86:686a.
30. Tepler I, Elias L, Smith JW II, et al. A randomized placebo-controlled trial of recombinant human interleukin-11 in cancer patients with severe thrombocytopenia due to chemotherapy. Blood 1996;87:3607-14.
31. Wendling F, Varlet P, Charon M, Tambourin P. MPLV: A retrovirus complex inducing an acute myeloproliferative leukemic disorder in adult mice. Virology 1986;149(2):242-6.
32. Souyri M, Vigon I, Penciolelli JF, et al. A putative truncated cytokine receptor gene transduced by the myeloproliferative leukemia virus immortalizes hematopoietic progenitors. Cell 1990;63:1137-47.
33. Vigon I, Mornon JP, Cocault L, et al. Molecular cloning and characterization of MPL, the human homolog of the v-mpl oncogene: Identification of a member of the hematopoietic growth factor receptor superfamily. Proc Natl Acad Sci USA 1992;89:5640-4.
34. deSauvage FJ, Hass PE, Spencer SD, et al. Stimulation of megakaryocytopoiesis and thrombopoiesis by the c-*mpl* ligand. Nature 1994; 369:533-8.
35. Hunt P, Li YS, Nichol JL, et al. Purification and biologic characterization of plasma-derived megakaryocyte growth and development factor. Blood 1995;86(2):540-7.

36. Lok S, Kaushansky K, Holly RD, et al. Cloning and expression of murine thrombopoietin cDNA and stimulation of platelet production in vivo. Nature 1994;369(6481):565-8.
37. Ogami K, Shimada Y, Sohma Y, et al. The sequence of a rat cDNA encoding thrombopoietin. Gene 1995;158(2):309-10.
38. Kuter DJ, Rosenberg RD. Appearance of a megakaryocyte growth-promoting activity, megapoietin, during acute thrombocytopenia in the rabbit. Blood 1994;84(5):1464-72.
39. Wendling F, Maraskovsky E, Debili N, et al. c-*Mpl* ligand is a humoral regulator of megakaryocytopoiesis. Nature 1994;369:571-4.
40. Kaushansky K, Lok S, Holly RD, et al. Promotion of megakaryocyte progenitor expansion and differentiation by the c-*Mpl* ligand thrombopoietin. Nature 1994;369:568-71.
41. Lok S, Kaushansky K, Holly RD, et al. Cloning and expression of murine thrombopoietin cDNA and stimulation of platelet production in vivo. Nature 1994;369:565-8.
42. de Sauvage FJ, Hass PE, Spencer SD, et al. Stimulation of megakaryocytopoiesis and thrombopoiesis by the c-*Mpl* ligand. Nature 1994;369:533-8.
43. Kaushansky K, Broudy VC, Lin N, et al. Thrombopoietin, the Mp1 ligand, is essential for full megakaryocyte development. Proc Natl Acad Sci USA 1995;92:3234-8.
44. Foster DC, Sprecher CA, Grant FJ, et al. Human thrombopoietin: Gene structure, cDNA sequence, expression, and chromosomal localization. Proc Natl Acad Sci USA 1994; 91:13023-7.
45. Chang MS, McNinch J, Basu R, et al. Cloning and characterization of the human megakaryocyte growth and development factor (MGDF) gene. J Biol Chem 1995;270:511-4.
46. McCarty IM, Kaushansky K. Functional characterization of the thrombopoietin promoter (abstract). Blood 1995;86:364a.
47. Dorsch M, Fan PD, Bogenberger J, Goff SP. TPO and IL-3 induce overlapping but distinct protein tyrosine phosphorylation in a myeloid precursor cell line. Biochem Biophys Res Commun 1995;214:424-31.
48. Sasaki K, Odai H, Hanazono Y, et al. TPO/c-*mpl* ligand induces tyrosine phosphorylation of multiple cellular proteins including proto-oncogene products, Vav and c-Cbl, and Ras signaling molecules. Biochem Biophys Res Commun 1995;216:338-47.
49. Kaushansky K. The mpl ligand: Molecular and cellular biology of the critical regulator of megakaryocyte development. Stem Cells 1994; 12:91-6.

50. Lok S, Foster DC. The structure, biology and potential therapeutic applications of recombinant thrombopoietin. Stem Cells 1994;12:586-98.
51. Broudy VC, Lin NL, Kaushansky K. Thrombopoietin (c-*mpl* ligand) acts synergistically with erythropoietin, stem cell factor, and interleukin-11 to enhance murine megakaryocyte colony growth and increases megakaryocyte ploidy in vitro. Blood 1995;85:1719-26.
52. Debili N, Wendling F, Katz A, et al. The Mpl-ligand or thrombopoietin or megakaryocyte growth and differentiative factor has both direct proliferative and differentiative activities on human megakaryocyte progenitors. Blood 1995;86:2516-25.
53. Banu N, Wang JF, Deng B, et al. Modulation of megakaryocytopoiesis by thrombopoietin: the c-Mpl ligand. Blood 1995; 86:1331-8.
54. Kaushansky K, Broudy VC, Grossmann A, et al. Thrombopoietin expands erythroid progenitors, increases red cell production, and enhances erythroid recovery after myelosuppressive therapy. J Clin Invest 1995;96:1683-7.
55. Ault KA, Mitchell J, Knowles C. Recombinant human thrombopoietin augments spontaneous and ADP induced platelet activation both in vitro and in vivo (abstract). Blood 1995;86:367a.
56. Oda A, Miyakawa Y, Druker BJ, et al. Thrombopoietin primes human platelet aggregation induced by shear stress and by multiple agonists. Blood 1996;87(11):4664-70.
57. Kuter DJ, Rosenberg RD. The reciprocal relationship of thrombopoietin (c-*Mpl* ligand) to changes in the platelet mass during busulfan-induced thrombocytopenia in the rabbit. Blood 1995;85:2720-30.
58. Nichol J, Hornkohl A, Selesi D, et al. TPO levels in plasma of patients with thrombocytopenia or thrombocytosis (abstract). Blood 1995; 86:371a.
59. Emmons RVB, Shulman NR, Reid DM, et al. Thrombocytopenic patients with aplastic anemia have high TPO levels whereas those with immune thrombocytopenia are much lower (abstract). Blood 1995; 86:372a.
60. Gurney AL, Carver-Moore K, de Sauvage FJ, Moore MW. Thrombocytopenia in c-mpl-deficient mice. Science 1994;265:1445-7.
61. McCarty JM, Sprugel KH, Fox NE, et al. Murine thrombopoietin mRNA levels are modulated by platelet count. Blood 1995;86:3668-75.
62. Farese AM, Hunt P, Boone T, MacVittie TJ. Recombinant human megakaryocyte growth and development factor stimulates thrombocytopoiesis in normal nonhuman primates. Blood 1995;86:54-9.

63. Basser R, Clarke K, Fox R, et al. Randomized, double-blind, placebo-controlled phase I trial of PEG-ylated megakaryocyte growth and development factor (PEG-rHuMGDF) administered to patients with advanced cancer before and after chemotherapy—Early results (abstract). Blood 1995;86:257a
64. Begley G, Basser R, Clarke K, et al. Randomized, double-blind, placebo-controlled phase I trial of PEG-ylated megakaryocyte growth and development factor (PEG-rHuMGDF) administered to patients with advanced cancer before and after chemotherapy (abstract). Proc Annu Meet Am Soc Clin Oncol 1996;15:719
65. Rasko JEJ, Basser R, O'Malley CJ, et al. in vitro studies from a phase I randomized, blinded trial of PEG-ylated megakaryocyte growth and development factor (PEG-rHuMGDF) (abstract). Blood 1995;86:497a.
66. Fanucchi M, Glaspy J, Crawford J, et al. Safety and biologic efficacy of PEG-ylated megakaryocyte growth and development factor (PEG-rHuMGDF) in lung cancer patients receiving carboplatin and paclitaxel: Randomized placebo-controlled phase I study (abstract). Proc Annu Meet Am Soc Clin Oncol 1996;15:720.
67. Vadhan-Raj S, Burris H, Benjamin RS, et al. Single-dose therapy with recombinant human thrombopoietin (rhTPO) in patients receiving cytotoxic chemotherapy (abstract). J Clin Oncol 1996;14:1747.

In: Davenport RD, Snyder EL, eds.
Cytokines in Transfusion Medicine: A Primer
Bethesda, MD: AABB Press, 1997

8

Cytokines in Ex-Vivo Stimulation of Hematopoietic Progenitor Cells

STEPHEN G. EMERSON, MD, PhD

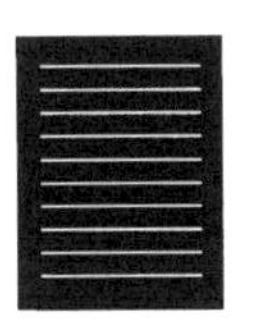

THE DEVELOPMENT OF THE CLINICAL PRACTICE OF hematology over the past several decades has exemplifed the dialectic application of both cellular therapies and molecular pharmacology. Initially, whole and then fractionated blood products were the sole "hemotherapy" that existed. The applicability of these blood products was limited by the natural life span of the products transfused: red blood cells lasted several weeks to months, immu-

Stephen G. Emerson, MD, PhD, Chief, Hematology-Oncology Division and Professor of Medicine and Pediatrics, University of Pennsylvania School of Medicine, Philadelphia, Pennsylvania

This work is supported by grants from the National Institutes of Health and the Leukemia Society of America. Dr. Emerson is a founder and consultant to Aastrom Biosciences, Inc., which has proprietary rights to perfusion-based hematopoietic culture technologies mentioned in this chapter. This chapter is modified and updated (with permission from WB Saunders, Inc.) from an article entitled "Ex vivo expansion of hematopoietic precursors, progenitors and stem cells: The next generation of cellular therapeutics," which appeared in Blood 1996;87:3082-8.

noglobulin fractions lasted days to weeks, platelets lasted a few days, and neutrophils lasted only a few hours.

A truly dramatic advance was made with the molecular cloning and in vivo application of human hematopoietic growth factors, or cytokines. Initially, these polypeptides were characterized by their activities on hematopoietic cell lines or on populations of normal hematopoietic cells. However, in pioneering studies by Donahue et al,[1] it was found that granulocyte-macrophage colony-stimulating factor (GM-CSF) had the same activity after injection into primates in vivo that it had on in-vitro hematopoietic cells, ie, it stimulated the differentiation, proliferation, and activation of neutrophils, monocyte-macrophages, and eosinophils. Similar studies with erythropoietin (EPO)[2] and granulocyte colony-stimulating factor (G-CSF) followed, and likewise demonstrated essentially identical activities in vivo to those found in preclinical in-vitro studies. This homeomorphism, combined with the relatively restricted activities of these three cytokines, has allowed for these cytokines to achieve worldwide clinical use as in-vivo pharmaceuticals.

When more complex, multifarious cytokines such as interleukin-3 (IL-3), interleukin-6 (IL-6), tumor necrocis factor-alpha (TNF-α), stem cell factor (SCF), and interleukin-1α (IL-1α) were studied in vivo, however, the results were not nearly as useful. In some cases, such as with IL-1α and TNF-α, patients suffered hemodynamic and generalized homeostatic symptoms above and beyond any beneficial hematopoietic effects. For others, such as SCF, differentiating and activating effects on mast cells proved to be so marked as to overshadow any positive hematopoietic effects, thereby making the product unsafe as a hematopoietic stimulant. Most puzzling of all, cytokines such as IL-3 and IL-6, which would be predicted to have major and useful properties as multilineage hematopoietic stimulants on the basis of in-vitro assays, were found to have surprisingly weak effects when administered in vivo.

Most recently, attention has therefore shifted to the combined application of hematopoietic cells cultured in vitro in the presence of hematopoietic cytokines. The hope is that the hematopoietic stimulatory capacity of multiple cytokines in vitro will be harnessed without nonhematopoietic side effects or suppressive feedback inhibition that might dampen their effects. After incubation, the stimulated cells can be washed to remove any remaining cytokines, and the ex-vivo cultured-activated expanded cell populations can be returned to the patient for clinical benefit. In this way, the hematopoietic effects of cytokines can be maximized without nonhematopoietic side effects.

This chapter briefly reviews the history of ex-vivo hematopoietic cultures. The roles of particular cytokines are highlighted, including those cytokines believed to be effective at the present time and those whose utility appears to be on the horizon. Finally, the initial experience with the delivery of ex-vivo expanded-activated human hematopoietic cells to patients is reviewed.

Short- and Long-Term Bone Marrow Culture

Three decades ago, Bradley and Metcalf[3] introduced a new semisolid culture system, the colony-forming assay, with several fascinating novel features. This assay directly identifies primitive hematopoietic cells in vitro by virtue of their progeny-forming focal colonies and visually display their dynamics and kinetics. These powerful features allow investigators to infer features to stem cell biology that were otherwise essentially invisible.

However, even in these first studies, a "Heisenberg perturbation" was created. The very act of aspirating and explanting the marrow so that its dynamics could be studied dramatically altered the biology that was observable. The most dramatic perturbation seen in colony assays is that hematopoiesis is only temporary, with proliferation seen only for 2-4 weeks, despite attempts to supplement the systems with nutrients and cytokines. This limitation shows that either the most primitive stem cells fail to survive and proliferate in these assays or that the cellular connection between the most primitive cells and truly proliferative progenitor cells is lost, so that the initial rapid production of precursors as progenitor-derived colonies is not sustained.

Attempts to mimic more closely stem cell biology ex vivo progressed to the development of liquid marrow culture systems by T.M. Dexter in the late 1970s.[4] In these "Dexter" cultures, the proliferation of stem cell-derived hematopoietic cells is dependent on the presence of an adherent layer, which represents a two-dimensional reconstitution of the mesenchymal interstitial component of marrow in vivo. These cells in the adherent layer exist in an organized, three-dimensional array in extremely close proximity to the developing hematopoietic cells.

Human marrow adaptations of Dexter cultures more clearly demonstrated the production kinetics of progenitors that had been observed in colony assays.[5] Like the colony assays, these cultures demonstrated the similar limitations that suggested that truly pluripotent stem cells do not survive or proliferate in these cultures. Whereas murine and tree shrew marrow cultures have been sustained for over one year, human Dexter cultures decay steadily from culture initiation and last only 6-12 weeks. More recently, limiting dilution techniques developed by Sutherland et al[6] have confirmed that the number of primitive cells capable of sustaining progenitor production begins to decline exponentially by 1 week in Dexter cultures. Similarly, Lansdorp et al,[7] through the use of cell surface phenotype analyses of human marrow cells in liquid culture, have found that primitive CD34+ CD38– cells fail to self-renew, at least when cultured in isolation from stromal cells.[7]

Two very different conclusions could be drawn from these experiments. First, it might be concluded that pluripotent stem cells have little, if any, potential for self-amplification. Under this scenario, hematopoiesis in vivo would be maintained by a succession of stem cells, which simply differentiate and extinguish. This conclusion, however, needs to be reconciled with the observations of Lemishka et al[8] and Abkowitz et al[9] who found that hematopoiesis in mice and cats appears to derive from a stable pool of stem cells for periods of over 6 months to years, respectively. Moreover, whereas hematopoiesis that is derived from more mature cells dies out, the stem cell pools that maintain such stable hematopoiesis do not extinguish. These data appear to be more consistent with a model in which the true number of long-lived stem cells is extremely low and that these cells initially divide very slowly. Thus, multilineage hematopoiesis is sustained temporarily, albeit for many months, by the terminal differentiation of cells that have already left the most primitive stem cell pool at the time of transplantation.

The alternative, more optimistic, conclusion that could be drawn from the limitations of liquid marrow cultures is that our efforts to culture hematopoietic cells ex vivo have failed to capture those elements of stem cell biology that occur in vivo and/or that could be maximized under ideal circumstances. Two distinctive approaches have been taken that pursue this more optimistic hypothesis: 1) liquid culture of purified primitive cells in high-dose recombinant cytokines, and 2) perfusion-based culture of whole marrow cell populations.

Current Approaches to Ex-Vivo Hematopoietic Expansion

Incubation of Selected CD34+ Cells with Combinations of High-Dose Cytokines

Incubation of selected CD34+ cells with combinations of high-dose cytokines has been the most commonly studied technique of ex-vivo hematopoietic culture. Haylock et al[10] first found that CD34+ mobilized peripheral blood cells that are highly purified by fluorescence immunocytometry could be driven to proliferate in a dilute culture in the presence of multiple hematopoietic growth factors. Under these conditions, the colony-forming unit–granulocyte macrophage (CFU-GM) pool expanded 20- to 60-fold over input over 14 days, and many more mature precursors were generated as well. These results have subsequently been reproduced by many other groups, including Srour et al,[11] Coutinho et al,[12] and Brugger et al[13] While there are some differences in the expansion protocols carried out by each group, they share the use of highly CD34+ selected cells, dilute culture conditions, and multiple high-dose cytokines. In these studies, CD34+ cell selection was implemented by precise but slower fluorescence-activated cell sorter (FACS) devices,[9,11] and by more rapid but less precise solid-phase immunoselection devices.[12,13] Without these features, proliferation is significantly reduced in these cultures. Similar results have been obtained from the use of marrow and umbilical cord blood cells with some interesting variations, as discussed below.

The results of these studies suggest that the presence of more mature, CD34– cells or their secreted metabolites may exert a strong suppressive effect on hematopoietic proliferation. Only by removing the CD34– cells and by culturing the remaining cells at low density can this inhibition be overcome, at least in static cultures in which all the cellular byproducts remain in the culture. The addition of high-dose cytokines, therefore, allows the proliferation and differentiation of many of the early preprogenitors present within the CD34+ population, thereby powerfully amplifying the progenitor and precursor pool.

Most of the progenitor cell amplification in these cultures appears to be occurring by terminal differentiation of preprogenitors and stem cells. Not only does the number of CD34+ cells themselves decline in these HDC cultures, but, the number of more primitive long-term culture-initiating cells (LT-CIC) rarely increases, and usually declines.[11-14] Thus, these cultures do not show evidence of true stem cell expansion, but rather powerful differentiation of a relatively early preprogenitor cell compartment. This loss of stem cells appears to be likely the result of the removal of stromal cells, which occurs during all current CD34 selection approaches whether implemented by FACS or solid-phase immunoselection devices.

Continuous Perfusion-Based Culture of Unselected Hematopoietic Cell Populations

The alternative approach to ex-vivo hematopoietic expansion is continuous perfusion-based culture of unselected hematopoietic cell populations. Perfusion, often used in conjunction with CSFs, is used to stimulate stromal cellular elements to support stem cell renewal and supply local proliferative and differentiative CSFs. Early studies by Caldwell et al[15,16] and Guba et al[17] demonstrated that rapid medium exchange stimulated the production of GM-CSF and IL-6 from bone marrow, stromal fibroblasts, and similar results have now been obtained for SCF. Schwartz et al[18,19] subsequently showed that similar rapid medium exchange schedules on whole marrow led to prolonged, stable progenitor cell production in culture, indicative of stem cell self-renewal. This effect was achieved by a combination of stimulation of the stromal elements and removal of metabolic byproducts produced by the maturing myeloid cells.

Taking advantage of stromal cell stimulation and added cytokines, rapid medium exchange has been combined recently with the addition of selected doses of exogenous CSFs. Koller et al[20] found that incubation of marrow mononuclear cells under continuous perfusion and oxygenation in the presence of low doses of SCF, IL-3, GM-CSF, and EPO result in a 10- to 20-fold expansion of total mononuclear cells and CFU-GM, along with a 4- to 8-fold expansion in LT-CIC. Subsequent studies by Koller et al[21] have shown that both the presence of the stromal layer, the presence of non-CD34+ nonstromal accessory cells, and the medium exchange provided by perfusion contribute to the maintenance and expansion of LT-CIC in these systems.[21] Sandstrom et al[22] found very similar results, demonstrating that perfusion strongly influences progenitor expansion and LT-CIC maintenance while CD34+ selection has no beneficial effects in and of itself. Recently, Zandstra et al[23] confirmed the effect of perfusion and cytokines in stimulating simultaneous LT-CIC and progenitor cell expansion in stroma-repleted bone marrow cells, demonstrating a several-fold expansion of LT-CIC in stirred flask bioreactors. Taken together, these studies suggest that ex vivo expansion of the progenitor cell pool concomitant with maintenance and limited expansion of the LT-CIC pool may be possible through a single-step culture of fairly unmanipulated marrow.

It is not known whether any of the currently employed human ex-vivo hematopoietic culture techniques support the amplification of the most primitive human hematopoietic stem cell pool. However, studies by Muench et al,[24] using murine marrow cells, showed that ex-vivo culture in the presence of SCF plus IL-1 reduced the number of transplanted cells required for radioprotection while simultaneously resulted in donor-derived hematopoiesis for over 1 year, including subsequent secondary transplantation. Thus, the only in-vivo experiments performed to date suggest that ex vivo culture may indeed support the survival and expansion of the long-term repopulating cell pool.

Similarly, it is not known precisely how many long-term repopulating cells are required for clinical transplantation. Extrapolating data from mice to humans suggests that at least 15,000 stem cells should be required for autologous transplants,[25] and perhaps 100-1000 times more for allogeneic transplants depending on the degree of genetic disparity between the donor and host. Whatever the precise number of stem cells, however, it seems clear that, despite preparative chemo- and/or radiotherapy, some threshold of long-lived stem cells must be provided to the transplant recipient, either via the graft or via survival of host stem cells. Given that the number of stem cells that might survive preparation will almost certainly vary widely among patients, it seems most prudent to attempt to provide hematopoietic infusions that contain the requisite number of long-term repopulating stem cells.

Sources of Hematopoietic Cells for Expansion

Marrow, mobilized peripheral blood, and umbilical cord blood have all been used successfully as starting populations for ex-vivo expansions. Each has its potential advantages and theoretical concerns as a clinical source.

Marrow

Marrow mononuclear cells in perfusion culture have been studied most extensively by Koller et al.[20,21] The advantage of this tissue is that pluripotent stem cells are known to be present at the start of the culture and all of the elements needed for their in vivo survival are likely to be present. In addition, the marrow cells in these studies have been put through little manipulation prior to culture. In fact, these cultures perform optimally when all marrow cellular elements are left in the starting cell population. While highly enriched CD34+ marrow cells can also be induced to proliferate in culture, progenitor and LT-CIC proliferation suffer comparably in the absence of the removed cell subsets. On the basis of numeric calculations, the results of these studies project that an engrafting dose of hematopoietic stem and progenitor cells could be obtained with approximately 5×10^8 marrow mononuclear cells, which could be obtained from a small number of analytic scale marrow aspirates in the outpatient setting.

Peripheral Blood

Mobilized peripheral blood CD34+ cells have been evaluated extensively by several groups[10-14] and show extremely high levels of progenitor and precursor cell expansion, with post-preexpansion progenitor cell ratios exceeding 50. The advantages of this approach are the availability of the starting material from circulating blood after patient mobilization with cytokines and/or chemotherapy and the excellent track record of mobilized peripheral blood for very rapid hematopoietic reconstitution. A significant potential concern with cultured mobilized peripheral blood CD34 cells is the long-term durability of the grafts in highly myeloablated patients because the survival of primitive hematopoietic cells in these cultures has been seen in only a few instances. However, many patients undergoing high-dose chemotherapy with hematopoietic cell rescue (autologous marrow transplantation) may be able to reconstitute long-term hematopoiesis from their residual, chemotherapy-treated marrow. If these patients can be reliably distinguished, then grafts depleted of true long-term repopulating cells might be quite sufficient.

Cord Blood

Umbilical cord blood (UCB) cells offer an increasingly intriguing approach to the application of ex vivo stem cell expansion to clinical hematology. Nearly a decade ago, Broxmeyer and colleagues[26] made fundamental and prescient observations on the composition of different hematopoietic compartments in human umbilical cord blood. They found that much like circulating adult peripheral blood, UCB contains clonogenic progenitor cells. However, the number of cells present is much higher in UCB (1-5/1000 mononuclear cells) than in adult peripheral blood (1-5/20,000). In addition, the progenitor-derived colonies observed were seen to be very large, including many macroscopic colonies.[27,28] These studies, which suggested that UCB contained a progenitor pool related to the primitive pool found in the fetal liver, were subsequently confirmed by many groups.

The observation that the colonies in cultured UCB were generally large and multifocal, combined with longstanding observations of Fleishman and Mintz[29] who demonstrated that fetal stem cells had a competitive repopulating advantage over adult stem cells,[29] suggested that UCB stem and progenitor cells might have higher proliferative capacity and perhaps higher capacity for self-renewal. Lu et al and Carow et al[30,31] recently demonstrated that this is indeed the case. These authors found that individual UCB-derived CFU-GEMM colonies could be replated 4 to 5 times, maintaining multilineage hematopoiesis, compared with adult CFU-GEMM colonies, which have little or no replating ability. In addition, Landsdorp et al[7,32] found that UCB CD34+ cells are able to generate several thousand more mature cells in culture without reducing the number of CD34+ cells in the culture. This is in contrast to adult marrow in which CD34+ cells decline rapidly in culture, indicating a loss of primitive self-renewing cells. Finally, studies by Moore[33] indicate that low density culture of UCB CD34+

cells can result in a more than 20-fold increase in primitive Δ cells, which is in contrast to similar cultures of adult marrow in which Δ cells rarely increase by even three-fold. These studies indicate that UCB progenitors have a greatly increased capacity to support the production of more mature cells and to self-renew, and suggest that UCB might be a superior source of stem and progenitor cells for clinical transplantation.

On the basis of these careful preclinical studies, UCB was first used as a source of transplantable stem cells in 1990 by Gluckman et al[34] for a child with Fanconi's Anemia. Overall, the results of the more than 65 UCB transplants to date suggest that: 1) UCB stem cells exist and can engraft after infusion, although engraftment kinetics are somewhat slower than for marrow or mobilized peripheral blood cells; and 2) recipient graft-vs-host disease is no more severe, and perhaps milder, with UCB cells than with marrow donor cells.[35-37] However, it is possible that the in-vivo expansion potential of UCB cells is not infinite, nor easily influenced after reinfusion. While some larger children weighing as much as 70 kg have successfully engrafted following UCB transplantation, a number of recipients weighing over 40 kg have failed to engraft following UCB infusions from standard cord blood collections. Therefore, successful ex-vivo expansion of UCB could have a tremendous impact on the applicability of UCB to diverse clinical settings involving the treatment of older children and adults. Current studies from several laboratories suggest that UCB progenitors and LT-CIC pools can be readily expanded, apparently to a greater extent than marrow or mobilized peripheral blood.[38-41]

Hematopoietic Growth Factors in the Ex-Vivo Expansion Cultures

Ex-vivo hematopoietic expansion cultures have been performed with a variety of combinations of cytokines, with only partial consensus emerging as to the optimal combination for clinical use. In general, those cytokines that either directly or synergistically stimulate the proliferation and differentiation of progenitors into recognizable precursor cells are also effective in stimulating the expansion of the progenitor cell compartment in liquid culture. For example, Haylock et al[10] found that the combination of IL-1β, IL-3, IL-6, G-CSF, GM-CSF, and SCF was superior to combinations lacking any one of these six cytokines. These findings have been reproduced by many groups, with the notable exception of Brugger and colleagues,[13] who found that the inclusion of G-CSF and/or GM-CSF in their cultures resulted in greater numbers of total cells, but lower numbers of clonogenic progenitor cells. In the case of whole marrow perfusion cultures, substantial quantities of IL-6 and IL-1 appear to be provided by the stromal and accessory cells, so that adding these cytokines has no additional beneficial effect.[17,42] The quantities of SCF and Flk-2 ligand produced by these cells appear to be fairly low, such that addition of SCF or Flk-2 ligand substantially increases the yield of progenitors recovered from perfusion-based marrow mononuclear cell cultures. Conversely, inclusion of macrophage inflammatory protein-1 alpha (MIP-1α), TNF-α, and transforming growth factor-beta (TGF-β) in most expansion cultures reported to date results in decreased progenitor cell and precursor cell yields.[43]

The survival and proliferation of more primitive preprogenitor cells may also be influenced by the cytokines that supplement the expansion cultures. This is particularly true of enriched CD34+ cell expansion cultures. Henschler et al[14] directly compared several combinations of cytokines using a cobblestone area-forming cell (CAFC) assay, which they have validated as correlating closely with "classical" LT-CIC assays. They have found that inclusion of only SCF, IL-3, or both, leads to substantial declines in CAFC over 12 days. Combinations of SCF and IL-3 plus either G-CSF, IL-1, or IL-6 prevent much of the loss, and simultaneous culture of SCF, IL-3, IL-1, IL-6, and EPO leads to approximate maintenance of LT-CIC during this period of time.[14] In perfusion-based cultures in which remaining stromal elements produce endogenous SCF, IL-6, and undoubtedly other cytokines, requirements for adding exogenous multiple cytokines for LT-CIC maintenance are not as stringent.

New Cytokines: Flk-2/Flt-3 Ligand and Thrombopoietin

Two recently cloned cytokines offer particular promise for additional application to human ex vivo hematopoietic cultures. Flk-2/Flt-3 ligand, originally cloned as the ligand for a protein tyrosine kinase whose expression within hematopoiesis is limited to primitive cells, appears to have potent effects on primitive cells of multiple hematopoietic lineages. In long-term hematopoietic cultures Flk-2/Flt-3 ligand augments and partially substitutes for the effects of stromal cells, allowing the persistence of hematopoietic cultures for many months. In addition, this cytokine appears to support preferentially the survival of primitive CD34+ CD38– cells in liquid cultures. Thus, it seems possible that additional studies will demonstrate an important role for Flk-2/Flt-3 ligand in the support of LT-CIC survival and expansion during ex-vivo culture, thus allowing efficient stem cell expansion and gene transfer.

Thrombopoietin

TPO has been cloned recently by expression as well, and its activity has been confirmed in animal and human studies in vivo.[44,45] The extremely high potency of TPO, with activities both at the level of committed megakaryocytic progenitors as well as more primitive multilineage progenitor cells, suggests that TPO may have extremely beneficial uses for the direct ex vivo production of platelets for in-vivo transfusion therapies. Additional studies with TPO in ex-vivo hematopoietic cultures are awaited with keen interest.

Initial Clinical Experience with Ex-Vivo Expanded Hematopoietic Cells

Cultured, human, hematopoietic cells have been studied in clinical settings for several years. Following promising preliminary experiments in mice,[46] Dexter and colleagues first returned cultured marrow to two patients in 1983.[47] Their group has extended this approach over the years, particularly in patients with acute myelogenous leukemia. Barnett and colleagues[48] have extensive experience in returning cultured marrow to patients with chronic myelogenous leukemia.[48] Although these early transplants did not intentionally amplify the cultured cells, they demonstrated that this sort of process could be performed safely and that the reinfusion of proliferating cultured cells was not overtly toxic, although recovery of myelopoiesis in these patients was often quite delayed.

Silver et al[49] first returned marrow mononuclear cells derived from 14-day perfusion cultures supplemented with IL-3, GM-CSF, EPO, and SCF as adjuncts to autografts in five patients receiving cellular support for high-dose cancer therapy for Hodgkin's disease and non-Hodgkin's lymphoma. They found no toxicities associated with the infusions, and each of the patients had a benign posttransplant course. Six of the patients had either a single fever or no fevers. Neutrophil counts of 500/μL were reached in 8 - 15 days, and platelet independence was reached in 12-21 days. Champlin et al[50] recently reported a very similar experience with marrow mononuclear cells derived from 14-day perfusion cultures supplemented with EPO and the GM-CSF/IL-3 fusion protein PIXY321. In a study of nine patients undergoing autologous, bone marrow transplantation for breast cancer, all patients achieved neutrophil counts of more than 500/μL by day 10-13, and all sustained platelet counts of more than 25,000/μL by day 16.[50] More recently, Bender et al studied five patients who received enriched CD34+ mobilized peripheral blood cells cultured with PIXY321 for 12 days, infused the day after reinfusion of the standard, noncultured peripheral blood mononuclear cells dose. They found no toxicities associated with the infusions, and all five patients recovered neutropoiesis and megakaryocytopoiesis with kinetics at least as rapid as patients undergoing standard peripheral blood transplantation.[51] Thus, it appears that supplementation of standard marrow or peripheral blood autografts with either in vitro cultured marrow or peripheral blood mononuclear cells may well have the ability to support reproducible and prompt early neutrophil and platelet recovery, eliminating the worrisome problem of "outliers" with very delayed hematopoietic recoveries.

Brugger et al[52] have returned ex-vivo cultured mobilized peripheral blood cells alone to patients undergoing high-dose, although not truly myeloablative, chemotherapy, with exciting and encouraging early results. Fifteen million CD34+ mobilized peripheral blood cells were cultured in the presence of SCF, IL-1β, IL-3, IL-6, and EPO for 12 days. The cells resulting from this culture were returned either as supplements to a standard mobilized peripheral blood reinfusion (four patients) or as sole myeloprotective support (six patients). Of the six patients who received ex-vivo cultured cells alone, five survived and engrafted promptly. Mean neutrophil recoveries to 500/μL and 1000/μL absolute neutrophil count occurred 2 days later than in patients receiving both native and cultured cells, while platelet recoveries were indistinguishable in the two small groups. Interestingly, these authors found that there was a strong correlation between the number of expanded cells that were returned to the patients and the rapidity of platelet recovery, a correlation also observed in the original patients studied by Silver et al.[49] Overall, while it is too early to know the durability of the hematopoietic recoveries in these patients, and while the chemotherapy regimen employed may not have been truly myeloablative, these results clearly support the notion that a fairly small number of enriched hematopoietic progenitor cells cultured ex vivo under these conditions will initiate hematologic reconstitution.

However, more recent reports suggest that the recoveries engendered by these cultured cells may not be durable. Holyoake et al[53] recently reported the failure of ex vivo, stromal-free cultured CD34+ cells to support hematopoiesis durably following intensive chemotherapy.[53] These results suggest that the activities of the ex-vivo cultured cells may be restricted by the presence or absence of primitive, proliferative hematopoietic stem cells within the cell populations. Thus, it is possible that the application of simply differentiating high-dose cytokine cultures, which make no effort to retain stem cells, may be limited.

Table 8-1. Potential Clinical Application of Ex-Vivo Expanded Hematopoietic Cells

Myelopoietic Support of a Hematopoietically Compromised Host
- Autologous bone marrow transplantation
- Allogeneic bone marrow transplantation
- Nontransplant nadir rescue
- Umbilical cord blood transplantation

Ex-Vivo Education/Modification of Stem Cells and Derivative Cells
- T-cell depletion of stem cell grafts for allogeneic bone marrow transplantation
- Active purging of tumor cells from stem cell autografts in vitro
- Adoptive immunotherapy via T-cells generated and educated ex vivo
- Permanent genetic modification of stem cells

Potential Clinical Uses for Ex-Vivo Expanded Hematopoietic Cells

With full command over hematopoietic cell expansion and differentiation, a wide array of clinical applications can be envisioned (Table 8-1). At the most basic level, ex-vivo expanded myeloid cells could have utility in hematopoietically compromised patients in a variety of settings now commonly seen in clinical hematology/oncology, including high-dose chemotherapy and autologous and allogeneic bone marrow transplantation. In the case of transplantation, ex-vivo expansion can be employed to reduce the morbidity of the induced nadirs and to eliminate the need for operative harvests or leukapheresis procedures. For autologous applications, ex-vivo cultures and expansions could theoretically be employed for directed tumor purging, both passive purging in culture and active, specific antitumor therapeutics.

A direct extension of the myeloid expansion approach would be to use ex-vivo expanded UCB for hematopoietic support. This approach is intriguing for several reasons. First, it is clear that fetal and umbilical cord hematopoietic cells have an increased proliferative capacity, and it may be the case that fetal and umbilical cord stem cells have increased capacity for true self-renewal. Second, there is the possibility, though not yet the evidence, that lymphoid cells derived from umbilical stem cells may cause less graft-vs-host disease in the allogeneic setting than do postnatal-derived lymphoid cells. Third, cord blood cells are truly a wasted resource waiting for medical application since they are simply discarded at the present time. Ex-vivo expansion will be very important for the general applicability of UCB to provide sufficient numbers of hematopoietic cells routinely for large recipients, whether UCB is used either in the form of a large matched-unrelated donor bank, or as long-term autologous hematopoietic "insurance."

The ability to control hematopoietic expansion beyond the myeloid lineage could have wider and more sophisticated applications. Ex-vivo lymphoid expansion from prolymphocytes could allow one to perform ex vivo education of donor T cells to antitumor activity. This could provide a more sustained and effective approach to adoptive immunotherapy, such as lymphokine-activated killer cell therapy. One could envision the simultaneous expansion of myeloid and lymphoid cells prior to reinfusion, thereby providing both myeloid support and direct, expanded antitumor activities.

Finally, the ability to control and amplify pluripotent stem cell self-renewal and expansion will provide a major boon to stem cell gene therapeutics. For both retrovirus and adenovirus-based vectors, stem cell division appears to be a major rate-limiting step to stem cell transduction. The ability to regulate stem cell division ex vivo would permit increased levels of stem cell transduction, thus allowing diverse applications of stem cell modification. Early applications of perfusion-based hematopoietic cell expansion techniques to retrovirus transduction suggest that this approach may indeed offer substantial promise for increased infection efficiency in primitive cells.[54]

Critical Experimental Questions—The Immediate Future

We are now in possession of only partial knowledge about the biology and applicability of ex-vivo hematopoiesis to clinical practice. However, the hematology community is now well positioned to ask and answer carefully the critical outstanding questions (Table 8-2): 1) Which patients will benefit, in an augmentation setting, from infused ex-vivo expanded cells? Autologous, allogenic, peripheral blood progenitor cell transplantation, nontransplant nadir reduction? 2) Does permanent reconstitution following autologous transplantation require LT-CIC, or are progenitors sufficient? Ever? Sometimes? Always? 3) Do ex-vivo expanded cells contain truly permanent repopulating stem cells suitable for allogeneic marrow transplantation (6 months? 2 years? more?)? 4) Will ex-vivo cultured stimulated marrow cells support hematopoietic reconstitution with the same rapidity as mobilized peripheral blood? 5) Why do UCB grafts take

Table 8-2. Hematopoietic Cytokines in Ex-Vivo Cell Culture

Cytokines
Cytokines that are Effective in Differentiating Primitive Cells for the Production of Late Progenitors and Precursors
Granulocyte colony-stimulating factor
Erythropoietin
Stem cell factor
Interleukin-3
Interleukin-6
Granulocyte-macrophage colony-stimulating factor
Interferon-γ
Thrombopoietin
Cytokines That May be Effective in Sustaining Primitive Hematopoietic Cells
Flk-2/Flt-3 ligand
Thrombopoietin
Stromal cells

slowly? Can ex-vivo expanded UCB cells circumvent this problem, or will the problem be accentuated in ex-vivo expanded grafts? 6) What is the in vivo physiology of T cells derived from ex-vivo cultured hematopoietic stem cells following transplantation?

Summary

Given these developments and opportunities, there will be an explosion in studies of ex-vivo expanded hematopoietic cells in the next few years. Autologous and allogeneic marrow transplantation augmentation and replacement, and high-dose chemotherapy support will likely be the initial applications. Studies examining the UCB expansion of hematopoietic cells to reduce the required amount of UCB needed for transplants in pediatric patients and to permit adult engraftment will likely follow. Simultaneous genetic modification and expansion of stem cells will also be explored in great detail. Overall, this promises to be an extremely exciting time in clinically applied hematopoiesis research. Major clinical benefits will likely result from our increasing ability to gain true control over the fate of hematopoietic stem cells ex vivo.

Acknowledgments

The author would like to thank Michael Clarke, MD; Bernhard Palsson, MD; Manfred Koller, MD; Sam Silver, MD; and Douglas Armstrong, MD, for many valuable discussions and insights. The secretarial and administrative support of Ms. Diane Meredith is also greatly appreciated.

References

1. Donahue RE, Wang EA, Stone DK, et al. Stimulation of haematopoiesis in primates by continuous infusion of recombinant human GM-CSF. Nature 1986;321:872-5.
2. Eschbach JW, Egrie JC, Downing MR, et al. Correction of the anemia of end-stage renal disease with recombinant human erythropoietin. N Engl J Med 1987;316:73-8.
3. Bradley TR, Metcalf D. The growth of mouse bone marrow cells in vitro. Aust J Exp Biol Med Sci 1966;44:287-97.
4. Dexter TM, Allen TD, Lajtha LG. Conditions controlling the proliferation of haemopoietic stem cells in vitro. J Cell Physiol 1977;91:335-46.
5. Gartner S, Kaplan HS. Long term culture of human bone marrow cells. Proc Natl Acad Sci USA 1980;74:4656-9.
6. Sutherland HJ, Hogge DE, Cook D, et al. Alternative mechanisms with and without steel factor support primitive human hematopoiesis. Blood 1993;81:1465-74.
7. Lansdorp PM, Dragowska W, Mayani H. Ontogeny-related changes in proliferative potential of human hematopoietic cells. J Exp Med 1993;178:787-95.
8. Lemishka I, Raulet DH, Mulligan RC. Developmental potential and dynamic behavior of hematopoietic stem cells. Cell 1986;45:917-27.
9. Abkowitz JL, Persik MT, Shelton GH, et al. Behavior of hematopoietic stem cells in a large animal. Proc Natl Acad Sci USA 1995;92:2031-5.
10. Haylock DN, To LB, Dowse TL, et al. Ex vivo expansion and maturation of peripheral blood CD34+ cells into the myeloid lineage. Blood 1992;80:1405-12.
11. Srour EG, Brandt JE, Briddell RA, et al. Long-term generation and expansion of human primitive hematopoietic progenitor cells in vitro. Blood 1993;81:661-9.
12. Coutinho LH, Will A, Radford J, et al. Effects of recombinant human granulocyte colony-stimulating factor (CSF), human granulocyte

macrophage-CSF, and gibbon interleukin-3 on hematopoiesis in human long-term bone marrow culture. Blood 1990;75:2118-29.
13. Brugger W, Mocklin W, Heimfeld S, et al. Ex vivo expansion of enriched peripheral blood CD34+ progenitor cells by stem cell factor, interleukin 1β (IL-1β), Il-6, Il-3, interferon-g and erythropoietin. Blood 1993;81:2579-84.
14. Henschler R, Brugger W, Luft T, et al. Maintenance of transplantation potential in ex vivo expanded CD34+-selected human peripheral blood progenitor cells. Blood 1994;84:2898-903.
15. Caldwell J, Locey B, Palsson BO, Emerson SG. The influence of culture perfusion conditions on normal human bone marrow stromal cell metabolism. J Cell Physiol 1991;147:344-53.
16. Caldwell J, Locey B, Clarke MF, et al. The influence of culture conditions on genetically engineered NIH-3T3 cells. Biotech Prog 1991;7:1-8.
17. Guba SC, Sartor CI, Gottschalk LR, et al. Bone marrow stromal cells secrete IL-6 and GM-CSF in the absence of inflammatory stimuli: Demonstration by serum-free bioassay, ELISA, and reverse transcriptase polymerase chain reaction. Blood 1992;80:1190-8.
18. Schwartz R, Palsson BO, Emerson SG. Rapid medium and serum exchange increases the longevity and productivity of human bone marrow cultures. Proc Natl Acad Sci USA 1991;88:6760-4.
19. Schwartz R, Emerson SG, Clarke MF, Palsson BO. in vitro myelopoiesis stimulated by rapid medium exchange and supplementation with hematopoietic growth factors. Blood 1991;78:3155-61.
20. Koller MR, Emerson SG, Palsson BO. Large-scale expansion of human hematopoietic stem and progenitor cells from bone marrow mononuclear cells in continuous perfusion culture. Blood 1993;82:378-84.
21. Koller MR, Palsson MA, Manchel I, Palsson BO. Long-term culture-initiating cell expansion is dependent on frequent medium exchange combined with stromal and other accessory cell effects. Blood 1995; 86:1784-93.
22. Sandstrom CE, Bender JG, Papoutsakis ET, Miller WM. Effects of CD34+ cell selection and perfusion on ex vivo expansion of peripheral blood mononuclear cells. Blood 1995;86:958-70.
23. Zandstra PW, Eaves CJ, Cameron C, Piret JM. Cytokine depletion in long-term stirred suspension cultures of normal human marrow. J Hematother 1995;4:235-45.
24. Muench MO, Firpo MT, Moore MAS. Bone marrow transplantation with Interleukin-1 plus kit-ligand ex vivo expanded bone marrow ac-

celerates hematopoietic reconstitution in mice without the loss of stem cell lineage and proliferative potential. Blood 1993;81:3463-73.
25. Spangrude GJ, Brooks DM, Tumas DB. Long-term repopulation of irradiated mice with limiting numbers of purified hematopoietic stem cells: In vivo expansion of stem cell phenotype but not function. Blood 1995;85:1006-16.
26. Broxmeyer HE, Douglas GW, Hangoc G, et al. Human umbilical cord blood as a potential source of transplantable hematopoietic stem/progenitor cells. Proc Natl Acad Sci USA 1989;86:3828-32.
27. Broxmeyer HE, Hangoc G, Cooper S, et al. Growth characteristics and expansion of human umbilical cord blood and estimation of its potential for transplantation in adults. Proc Natl Acad Sci USA 1992; 89:4109-13.
28. Broxmeyer HE, Kurtzberg J, Gluckman E, et al. Umbilical cord blood hematopoietic stem and repopulating cells in human clinical transplantation. Blood Cells 1991;17:313-29.
29. Fleischman RA, Mintz B. Development of adult bone marrow stem cells in H-2-compatible and -incompatible mouse fetuses. J Exp Med 1984;159:731-45.
30. Lu L, Xiao M, Shen RN, et al. Enrichment, characterization, and responsiveness of single primitive CD34 human umbilical cord blood hematopoietic progenitors with high proliferative and replating potential. Blood 1993;81:41-8.
31. Carow CE, Hangoc G, Broxmeyer HE. Human multipotential progenitor cells (CFU-GEMM) have extensive replating capacity for secondary CFU-GEMM: An effect enhanced by cord blood plasma. Blood 1993;81:942-9.
32. Mayani H, Lansdorp PM. Thy-1 expression is linked to functional properties of primitive hematopoietic progenitor cells from human umbilical cord blood. Blood 1994;83:2410-7.
33. Moore MAS. Ex vivo expansion and gene therapy using cord blood CD34+ cells. J Hematother 1993;2:221-4.
34. Gluckman E, Devergie A, Bourdeau-Esperou H, et al. Transplantation of umbilical cord blood in Fanconi's anemia. Nouv Rev Fr Hematol 1990;32:423-35.
35. Broxmeyer HE, Srivastava A, Lu L, et al. Cord blood transplantation: An update. Exp Hematol 1994;22:677-88.
36. Gluckman E, Broxmeyer HE, Auerbach AD, et al. Hematopoietic reconstitution in a patient with Fanconi's anemia by means of umbilical-

cord blood from an HLA-identical sibling. N Engl J Med 1989; 321:1174-8.

37. Wagner JE, Kernan, NA, Steinbuch M, et al. Allogeneic sibling umbilical-cord-blood transplantation in children with malignant and non-malignant disease. Lancet 1995;346:214-9.
38. Van Zant G, Rummel S, Koller MR, et al. Expansion in bioreactors of human hematopoietic progenitor populations from cord blood and mobilized peripheral blood. Blood Cells 1994;20:482-91.
39. Xiao M, Broxmeyer HE, Horie M, et al. Extensive proliferative capacity of single isolated CD34+ human cord blood cells in suspension culture. Blood Cells 1994;20:455-67.
40. Moore MAS, Hoskins I. Ex vivo expansion of cord blood-derived stem cells and progenitors. Blood Cells 1994;20:468-81.
41. Van Epps DE, Bender J, Lee W, et al. Harvesting, characterization and culture of CD34+ cells from human bone marrow, peripheral, and cord blood. Blood Cells 1994;20:411-23.
42. Koller MR, Bradley MS, Palsson BO. Growth factor consumption and production in perfusion cultures of human bone marrow correlate with specific cell production. Exp Hematol 1995;23:1275-83.
43. Mayani H, Little MT, Dragowska W, et al. Differential effects of the hematopoietic inhibitors MIP-1α, TGF-β, and TNF-α on cytokine-induced proliferation of subpopulations of CD34+ cells purified from cord blood and fetal liver. Exp Hematol 1995;23:422-7.
44. Lok S, Kaushansky K, Holly RD, et al. Cloning and expression of murine thrombopoietin cDNA and stimulation of platelet production in vivo. Nature 1994;369:565-8.
45. Kaushansky K, Lok S, Holly RD, et al. Promotion of megakaryocyte progenitor expansion and differentiation by the c-Mpl ligand thrombopoietin. Nature 1994;369:568-71.
46. Spooncer E, Dexter TM. Transplantation of long term cultured bone marrow cells. Transplantation 1984;35:624-7.
47. Chang J, Morgenstern G, Deakin D, et al. Reconstitution of haemopoietic system with autologous marrow taken during relapse of acute myeloblastic leukaemia and grown in long-term culture. Lancet 1986; 1:194-5.
48. Barnett MJ, Eaves CJ, Phillips GL, et al. Successful autografting in chronic myeloid leukaemia after maintenance of marrow in culture. Bone Marrow Transplant 1989;4:345-51.
49. Silver SM, Adams PT, Hutchinson RJ, et al. Phase I evaluation of ex vivo expanded hematopoietic cells produced by perfusion cultures in

autologous bone marrow transplantation(BMT) (abstract). Blood 1993;(Suppl 1)82:297a.

50. Champlin R, Mehra R, Gajewski J, et al. Ex vivo expanded progenitor cell transplantation in patients with breast cancer (abstract). Blood 1995;86(Suppl 1):295a.
51. Zimmerman TM, Bender JG, Lee WJ, et al. Large-scale selection of CD34+ peripheral blood progenitors and expansion of neutrophil precursors for clinical applications. J Hematother 1996;5:247-53.
52. Brugger W, Heimfeld S, Berenson RJ, et al. Reconstitution of hematopoiesis after high-dose chemotherapy by autologous progenitor cells generated ex vivo. N Engl J Med 1995;333:283-7.
53. Holyoake TL, Alcorn MJ, Richmond L, et al. A phase I study to evaluate the safety of re-infusing CD34+ cells expanded ex vivo as part or all of a PBPC transplant procedure (abstract). Blood 1995;86(Suppl 1):294a.
54. Eipers PG, Krause, JC, Palsson BO, et al. Retroviral infection of primitive hematopoietic cells in continuous perfusion culture. Blood 1995; 86:3754-62.

Index

Italicized page numbers indicate tables or figures.

C

R

S

T-V